This publication is intended to provide educational information for the reader on the covered subjects. It is not intended to take the place of personalized medical counseling, diagnosis, and treatment from a trained healthcare professional.

ISBN 978-1-998740-03-1 (Paperback)
ISBN 978-1-998740-04-8 (eBook)

Printed and bound in USA
Published by Loons Press

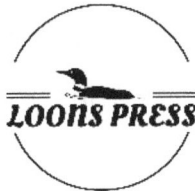

LOONS PRESS

Table Of Contents

How To Prevent Coronary Artery Disease

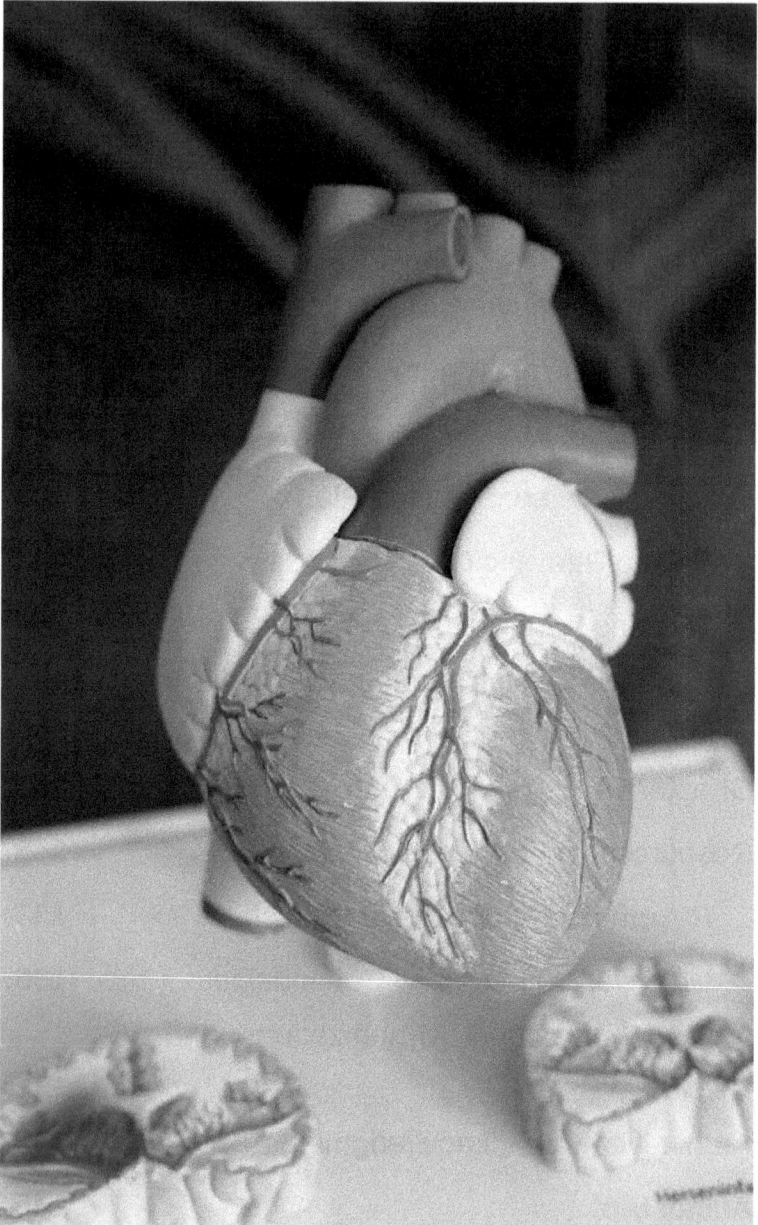

Chapter 1

Understanding Coronary Artery Disease

What is Coronary Artery Disease?

Coronary artery disease (CAD) is a progressive condition characterized by the narrowing or blockage of the coronary arteries, which supply oxygen-rich blood to the heart muscle.

This narrowing is typically caused by a process known as atherosclerosis, where fatty deposits, known as plaques, accumulate on the arterial walls.

Over time, these plaques can harden and narrow the arteries, leading to reduced blood flow to the heart. Understanding CAD is essential for prevention, as recognizing risk factors and symptoms can empower individuals to take proactive measures to protect their heart health.

The primary risk factors for coronary artery disease include high cholesterol levels, hypertension, smoking, obesity, and a sedentary lifestyle. Genetics also play a significant role, as a family history of heart disease can increase an individual's risk.

Furthermore, conditions such as diabetes and metabolic syndrome can exacerbate the development of CAD. Awareness of these factors is crucial, as many of them are modifiable through lifestyle changes, making prevention a realistic goal for many individuals.

Symptoms of coronary artery disease can vary widely, with some people experiencing no noticeable signs until a significant blockage occurs. Common symptoms include chest pain, often referred to as angina, which may radiate to the arms, back, or jaw.

Other signs may include shortness of breath, fatigue, and palpitations. In some cases, a heart attack may be the first indication of CAD, underscoring the importance of regular check-ups and monitoring heart health, particularly for those at higher risk.

Diagnosis of coronary artery disease typically involves a combination of medical history assessment, physical examinations, and diagnostic tests such as electrocardiograms, stress tests, and imaging studies. These evaluations help determine the severity of the disease and guide treatment options.

Early diagnosis is vital, as it opens up the opportunity for effective interventions that can halt or even reverse the progression of the disease through lifestyle adjustments and medical therapies.

Preventing coronary artery disease is achievable through a multifaceted approach that includes adopting a heart-healthy diet, engaging in regular physical activity, maintaining a healthy weight, and avoiding tobacco use. Additionally, managing stress levels and regular health screenings can further mitigate risks.

Education and awareness are key components in this prevention strategy, as individuals equipped with knowledge about CAD can make informed decisions that lead to improved heart health and overall well-being.

Risk Factors for Coronary Artery Disease

Coronary artery disease (CAD) is a leading cause of morbidity and mortality worldwide. Understanding the risk factors associated with CAD is essential for prevention. Various elements contribute to the development of this condition, and recognizing them can empower individuals to take proactive steps toward maintaining heart health. By identifying these risk factors, individuals can make informed lifestyle choices that may significantly reduce their chances of developing CAD.

One of the primary risk factors for coronary artery disease is age. As individuals grow older, the likelihood of experiencing CAD increases due to natural changes in the arteries and the cumulative effects of various risk factors over time. Men are generally at a higher risk at a younger age compared to women, although post-menopausal women catch up in risk levels.

Understanding the impact of age can help individuals prioritize heart health from an early age, emphasizing the importance of regular screenings and healthy lifestyle choices throughout their lives.

Another significant risk factor is the presence of high cholesterol levels. Low-density lipoprotein (LDL), often referred to as "bad" cholesterol, can accumulate in the walls of arteries, leading to atherosclerosis, which narrows and hardens the arteries.

Conversely, high levels of high-density lipoprotein (HDL), or "good" cholesterol, can help protect against CAD. Regular cholesterol screenings and dietary adjustments that promote healthy cholesterol levels are crucial steps in preventing coronary artery disease.

Hypertension, or high blood pressure, is also a critical risk factor for CAD. Elevated blood pressure strains the heart and can cause damage to the arteries over time.

Individuals with hypertension are encouraged to monitor their blood pressure regularly and adopt lifestyle modifications such as reducing sodium intake, maintaining a healthy weight, and engaging in regular physical activity. These changes can significantly lower blood pressure and reduce the risk of developing coronary artery disease.

Lifestyle choices play a pivotal role in the risk of coronary artery disease. Factors such as smoking, physical inactivity, and poor dietary habits contribute significantly to the development of CAD. Smoking damages blood vessels and accelerates the process of atherosclerosis, while a sedentary lifestyle can lead to obesity and increased cholesterol levels.

A diet high in saturated fats, trans fats, and sugars can also elevate the risk. By adopting a balanced diet rich in fruits, vegetables, whole grains, and lean proteins, along with regular exercise, individuals can effectively mitigate these lifestyle-related risk factors and promote cardiovascular health.

Symptoms and Diagnosis

Coronary artery disease (CAD) often develops gradually and may not present noticeable symptoms in its early stages. However, as the condition progresses, individuals may begin to experience a range of symptoms that can signal the presence of heart problems.

Common symptoms include chest pain or discomfort, often described as a feeling of pressure, squeezing, or fullness. This sensation may occur during physical activity or emotional stress and can sometimes be mistaken for indigestion. Recognizing these symptoms is crucial, as they can serve as early warning signs of CAD and prompt individuals to seek medical evaluation.

In addition to chest pain, other symptoms of coronary artery disease may include shortness of breath, fatigue, and lightheadedness. Shortness of breath can occur during exertion or even while at rest, depending on the severity of the disease. Fatigue may be disproportionate to the level of activity undertaken, indicating that the heart is not receiving adequate oxygen due to narrowed arteries.

Lightheadedness or dizziness can occur, particularly if the heart is struggling to pump blood effectively. Individuals experiencing these symptoms should not ignore them, as they may indicate the need for further assessment and intervention.

The diagnosis of coronary artery disease typically begins with a thorough medical history and physical examination conducted by a healthcare provider. The provider will inquire about the patient's symptoms, risk factors, and family history of heart disease.

This initial evaluation is crucial for identifying individuals who may be at higher risk for CAD. Depending on the findings from the physical examination and patient history, further diagnostic tests may be recommended to assess heart health more comprehensively.

Common diagnostic tests for coronary artery disease include electrocardiograms (ECGs), stress tests, and imaging studies such as echocardiograms or coronary angiography.

An ECG measures the electrical activity of the heart and can reveal irregularities that may suggest CAD. Stress tests help determine how the heart performs under physical stress, providing insight into its function.

Coronary angiography, often regarded as the gold standard for diagnosing CAD, involves the use of contrast dye to visualize the arteries and identify any blockages. These tests collectively provide valuable information that aids in diagnosing CAD and determining the appropriate course of action.

Early diagnosis and intervention are vital in managing coronary artery disease effectively. Individuals who recognize their symptoms and seek timely medical evaluation can significantly improve their heart health outcomes.

By understanding the signs of CAD and the diagnostic processes involved, individuals can take proactive steps toward prevention and management. This knowledge empowers them to work closely with healthcare providers to develop a personalized plan that may include lifestyle modifications, medication, or other interventions aimed at reducing the risk of heart disease and promoting overall cardiovascular health.

How To Prevent Coronary Artery Disease

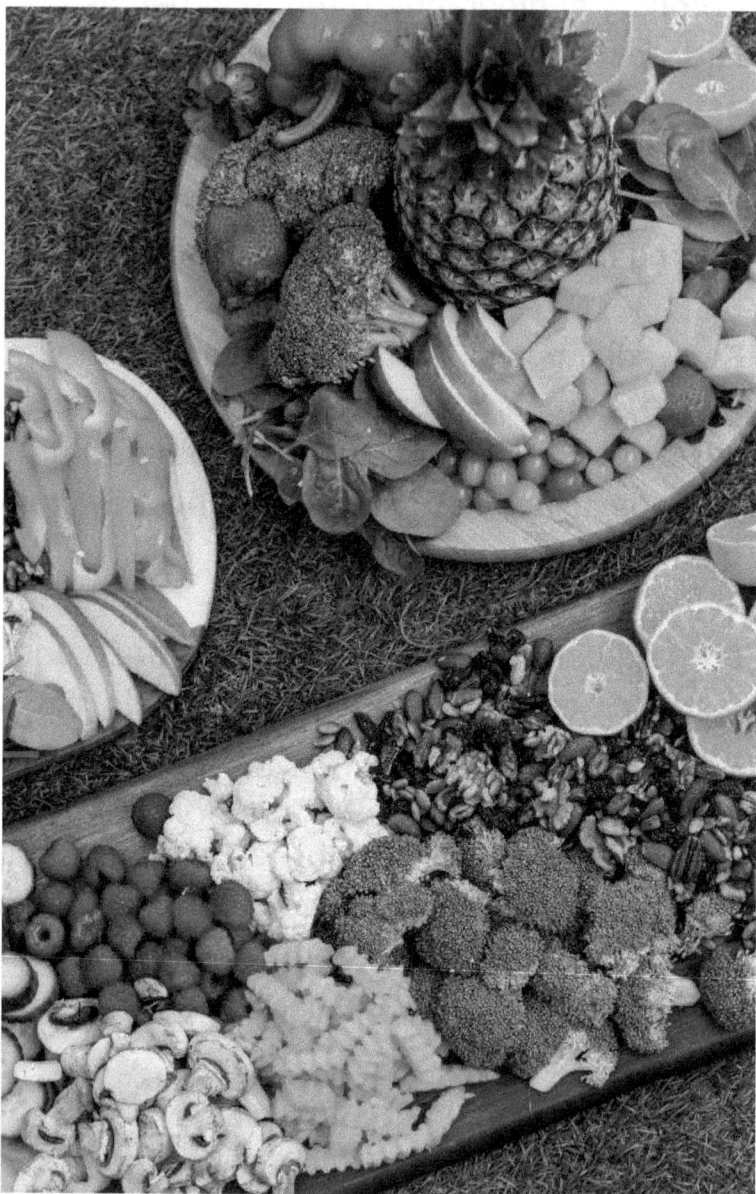

Chapter 2

The Role of Nutrition in Heart Health

Heart-Healthy Foods

Heart-healthy foods play a crucial role in the prevention of coronary artery disease (CAD), as they can help lower cholesterol levels, reduce blood pressure, and improve overall heart health.

A diet rich in specific nutrients can significantly impact the risk factors associated with CAD. Incorporating a variety of fruits, vegetables, whole grains, lean proteins, and healthy fats into daily meals can create a robust foundation for cardiovascular wellness.

Understanding the properties of these foods can empower individuals to make informed dietary choices that promote heart health.

Fruits and vegetables are essential components of a heart-healthy diet. They are packed with vitamins, minerals, and antioxidants that combat inflammation and oxidative stress, both of which can contribute to arterial damage. Leafy greens, berries, citrus fruits, and cruciferous vegetables like broccoli and cauliflower are particularly beneficial.

These foods are low in calories and high in fiber, which helps maintain a healthy weight and lowers cholesterol levels. Aim for a colorful variety to ensure a broad spectrum of nutrients, and consider incorporating them into every meal or as healthy snacks.

Whole grains provide another vital aspect of a heart-healthy eating plan. Foods such as oats, brown rice, quinoa, and whole wheat bread are rich in fiber that helps reduce the risk of developing high cholesterol. Fiber assists in the elimination of excess cholesterol from the body, and whole grains can also help regulate blood sugar levels.

Including at least three servings of whole grains in your daily diet can support heart health and contribute to overall well-being. When selecting grains, choose those that are minimally processed to maximize their health benefits.

Lean proteins are essential as well, especially for those looking to prevent CAD. Sources such as fish, poultry, beans, and legumes offer the necessary protein without excessive saturated fat found in red meats.

Fatty fish like salmon and mackerel are particularly beneficial due to their high omega-3 fatty acid content, which has been shown to reduce inflammation and lower the risk of heart disease. Incorporating plant-based proteins can also provide additional fiber and healthy nutrients.

A balanced intake of lean proteins can help maintain muscle mass and support metabolic health.

Healthy fats are another critical component of a heart-healthy diet. While it is essential to limit saturated and trans fats, incorporating sources of unsaturated fats can be advantageous. Foods such as avocados, nuts, seeds, and olive oil contribute to heart health by improving cholesterol levels and providing anti-inflammatory properties.

These fats can also aid in nutrient absorption and provide sustained energy. It is important to consume these fats in moderation and to focus on whole food sources rather than processed options. By prioritizing heart-healthy foods and making conscious dietary choices, individuals can significantly reduce their risk of coronary artery disease and enhance their overall health.

Dietary Patterns to Adopt

Adopting specific dietary patterns is crucial for individuals looking to prevent coronary artery disease. A heart-healthy diet emphasizes whole, minimally processed foods that promote cardiovascular health.

One of the most effective dietary approaches is the Mediterranean diet, which is rich in fruits, vegetables, whole grains, legumes, nuts, and healthy fats, particularly olive oil.

This pattern not only reduces the risk factors associated with coronary artery disease but also supports overall well-being. The inclusion of fish, especially fatty varieties like salmon and mackerel, provides essential omega-3 fatty acids that help lower triglyceride levels and reduce inflammation.

Another beneficial dietary pattern is the DASH (Dietary Approaches to Stop Hypertension) diet, designed to combat high blood pressure but also effective in promoting heart health. The DASH diet emphasizes the consumption of fruits, vegetables, low-fat dairy products, and whole grains while limiting saturated fat, cholesterol, and sodium.

This approach helps manage blood pressure and reduces the risk of developing coronary artery disease. By focusing on nutrient-dense foods, individuals can enhance their intake of potassium, calcium, and magnesium, which are vital for maintaining cardiovascular health.

Plant-based diets are increasingly recognized for their role in heart disease prevention. Adopting a vegetarian or vegan lifestyle can significantly lower the intake of saturated fats and cholesterol, typically found in animal products. Instead, these diets are rich in fibers, antioxidants, and phytochemicals that are protective against heart disease. Legumes, whole grains, fruits, and vegetables should form the foundation of a plant-based diet, ensuring that individuals receive adequate protein and essential nutrients while minimizing harmful fats.

In addition to specific dietary patterns, it is important to consider portion sizes and overall caloric intake. Mindful eating practices can help individuals become more aware of their dietary choices and prevent overconsumption.

By focusing on whole foods and minimizing processed and sugary items, individuals can create a balanced diet that supports heart health. Regularly incorporating a variety of foods also ensures a broad spectrum of nutrients, which is essential for maintaining optimal health and preventing coronary artery disease.

Lastly, hydration plays a vital role in overall health and should not be overlooked in dietary planning. Water is essential for various bodily functions, including nutrient transport and waste elimination. While beverages like sugary drinks and excessive alcohol can negatively impact heart health, opting for water, herbal teas, and other low-calorie beverages can promote hydration without added sugars.

By adopting these dietary patterns and making conscious food choices, individuals can significantly reduce their risk of coronary artery disease and enhance their overall quality of life.

Foods to Avoid

To effectively prevent coronary artery disease, it is crucial to be aware of the foods that can contribute to the development of this condition. Certain dietary choices, particularly those high in saturated fats, trans fats, and refined sugars, can lead to increased cholesterol levels and inflammation, both of which are risk factors for heart disease. By identifying and limiting these foods, individuals can take significant steps toward protecting their heart health.

One of the primary categories of foods to avoid includes processed and packaged snacks. These items often contain unhealthy trans fats, which are known to raise LDL cholesterol while lowering HDL cholesterol.

Common culprits include commercially baked goods, microwave popcorn, and various fried snacks. Instead of reaching for these convenient options, consider whole foods such as fruits, vegetables, nuts, and seeds, which provide essential nutrients without the harmful additives.

Another area of concern is red and processed meats, which have been linked to higher rates of heart disease. These meats are typically high in saturated fats and can contribute to arterial plaque buildup.

Processed meats, such as bacon, sausages, and deli meats, often contain additional preservatives and sodium, further exacerbating the risk factors for coronary artery disease. Opting for lean protein sources, such as fish, poultry, and plant-based proteins, can support heart health while providing necessary nutrients.

Sugary beverages and foods also pose significant risks. Sodas, energy drinks, and excessive consumption of sweets can lead to weight gain, insulin resistance, and increased triglyceride levels. These effects contribute to the development of coronary artery disease.

It is advisable to limit intake of sugary drinks and snacks and to replace them with water, herbal teas, or naturally sweetened alternatives. Focusing on whole fruits rather than fruit juices can also help reduce sugar intake while providing fiber and vitamins.

Lastly, it is important to be cautious with refined carbohydrates. Foods such as white bread, pastries, and many breakfast cereals can cause rapid spikes in blood sugar levels, leading to increased insulin production and potential weight gain.

These factors are associated with an elevated risk of heart disease. Choosing whole grain alternatives, which are higher in fiber and nutrients, can help maintain stable blood sugar levels and support overall cardiovascular health.

By being mindful of food choices and avoiding these harmful options, individuals can make significant strides in preventing coronary artery disease.

How To Prevent Coronary Artery Disease

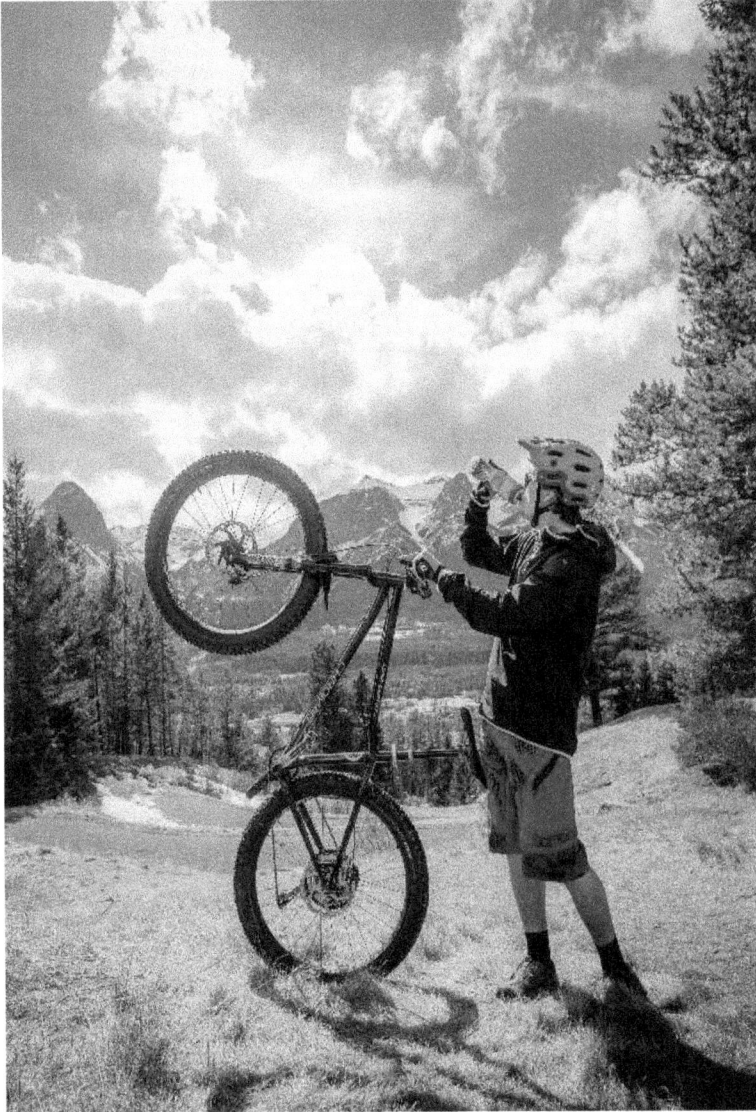

Chapter 3

The Importance of Physical Activity

Benefits of Regular Exercise

Regular exercise is a powerful tool in the fight against coronary artery disease (CAD). Engaging in physical activity helps to strengthen the heart muscle, improve blood circulation, and enhance overall cardiovascular health.

When blood flow is improved, the heart does not have to work as hard, reducing stress on the cardiovascular system. This decreased workload can lead to lower blood pressure and a reduced risk of developing heart-related issues.

One of the primary benefits of regular exercise is its ability to manage weight effectively. Maintaining a healthy weight is crucial for preventing CAD, as excess body weight can contribute to high cholesterol levels and elevated blood pressure.

Exercise burns calories and helps to build lean muscle mass, which can increase metabolism and promote fat loss. A combination of aerobic exercises, such as walking, cycling, or swimming, along with strength training, can significantly aid in achieving and maintaining a healthy weight.

Additionally, regular physical activity has been shown to improve lipid profiles by increasing high-density lipoprotein (HDL) cholesterol, commonly referred to as "good" cholesterol, while lowering low-density lipoprotein (LDL) cholesterol, or "bad" cholesterol.

This positive shift in cholesterol levels is vital for maintaining clear arteries and reducing the risk of plaque buildup that can lead to CAD. Incorporating moderate-intensity exercise into one's routine can lead to significant improvements in cholesterol levels over time.

Exercise also plays a crucial role in managing stress, which can be a contributing factor to heart disease. Physical activity triggers the release of endorphins, the body's natural mood lifters, which can help alleviate feelings of anxiety and depression.

Moreover, regular exercise promotes better sleep, which is essential for overall heart health. Reducing stress and improving sleep quality can lead to lower levels of cortisol, a hormone linked to increased heart disease risk when elevated for prolonged periods.

Finally, engaging in regular exercise fosters a sense of community and support when done in groups or classes. This social aspect can enhance motivation and accountability, making it easier to stick to an exercise routine. Building a support network of like-minded individuals who prioritize heart health can encourage lasting lifestyle changes.

By embracing regular physical activity, individuals not only bolster their cardiovascular health but also promote a holistic approach to well-being, significantly lowering the risk of coronary artery disease.

Recommended Types of Exercise

Incorporating regular exercise into your lifestyle is a crucial step in preventing coronary artery disease (CAD). Different types of physical activity can benefit cardiovascular health in unique ways.

Aerobic exercises, such as walking, jogging, cycling, and swimming, are particularly effective in enhancing heart health. Engaging in these activities increases your heart rate, improves blood circulation, and strengthens the heart muscle. Aim for at least 150 minutes of moderate-intensity aerobic exercise each week to significantly lower your risk of CAD.

Strength training is another essential component of a well-rounded exercise regimen. This type of exercise involves using weights or resistance bands to build muscle strength and endurance.

By increasing lean muscle mass, strength training helps improve metabolism and can contribute to weight management—an important factor in preventing CAD. It is recommended to perform strength training exercises at least two days a week, targeting all major muscle groups to achieve optimal benefits.

Flexibility and balance exercises are also important, particularly as you age. Activities such as yoga and tai chi not only enhance flexibility but also promote relaxation and reduce stress levels.

Stress management is vital for heart health, as chronic stress can contribute to high blood pressure and other risk factors associated with CAD. Incorporating flexibility and balance exercises into your routine can improve overall physical function and quality of life.

Interval training, which alternates periods of high-intensity exercise with lower-intensity recovery periods, has gained popularity for its efficiency and effectiveness. This approach can be applied to aerobic activities, such as cycling or running.

Studies have shown that interval training can lead to improved cardiovascular fitness and fat loss, making it a valuable addition to your exercise routine. However, it's important to approach interval training progressively, especially if you are new to exercising or have existing health concerns.

Lastly, it is essential to find an exercise routine that you enjoy and can commit to long-term. Consistency is key in reaping the benefits of physical activity for heart health.

Whether you prefer group classes, outdoor activities, or solo workouts, engaging in exercise that brings you joy will increase the likelihood of maintaining an active lifestyle.

Remember to consult with a healthcare professional before starting any new exercise program, especially if you have pre-existing health conditions or concerns related to coronary artery disease.

Creating an Exercise Routine

Creating an effective exercise routine is a crucial step in preventing coronary artery disease (CAD). Regular physical activity strengthens the heart muscle, improves blood circulation, and helps maintain a healthy weight, all of which contribute to better cardiovascular health. When designing an exercise routine, it is essential to consider various aspects such as frequency, intensity, duration, and type of exercise to ensure it aligns with personal health goals and physical capabilities.

The American Heart Association recommends that adults engage in at least 150 minutes of moderate-intensity aerobic exercise each week. This can be broken down into manageable sessions, such as 30 minutes of brisk walking five times a week.

For those who may find this daunting, starting with shorter sessions and gradually increasing duration can make the process more achievable. Consistency is key; thus, setting a regular schedule can help incorporate exercise into daily life, making it a habit rather than a chore.

In addition to aerobic activities, strength training should also be included in an exercise routine at least twice a week. This type of exercise helps to build muscle mass, which can enhance metabolic rate and improve overall body composition.

Bodyweight exercises, resistance bands, or free weights can all be effective methods for strength training. It is important to focus on major muscle groups while ensuring that the exercises are performed with proper form to prevent injury.

Flexibility and balance exercises also play an important role in a comprehensive exercise routine. Activities such as yoga or tai chi can improve flexibility, enhance balance, and reduce stress, all of which are beneficial for heart health. These practices can be incorporated into the routine on rest days or as part of a cool-down after more intense workouts. Maintaining flexibility and balance is particularly important as individuals age, as it can help prevent injuries and falls.

Lastly, it is advisable to consult with a healthcare professional before starting any new exercise program, especially for individuals with pre-existing health conditions or those who have been sedentary. A tailored exercise plan can ensure that the routine is safe and effective. Tracking progress through a journal or fitness app can also help maintain motivation and accountability.

By committing to a well-rounded exercise routine, individuals can significantly reduce their risk of coronary artery disease and improve their overall health and well-being.

How To Prevent Coronary Artery Disease

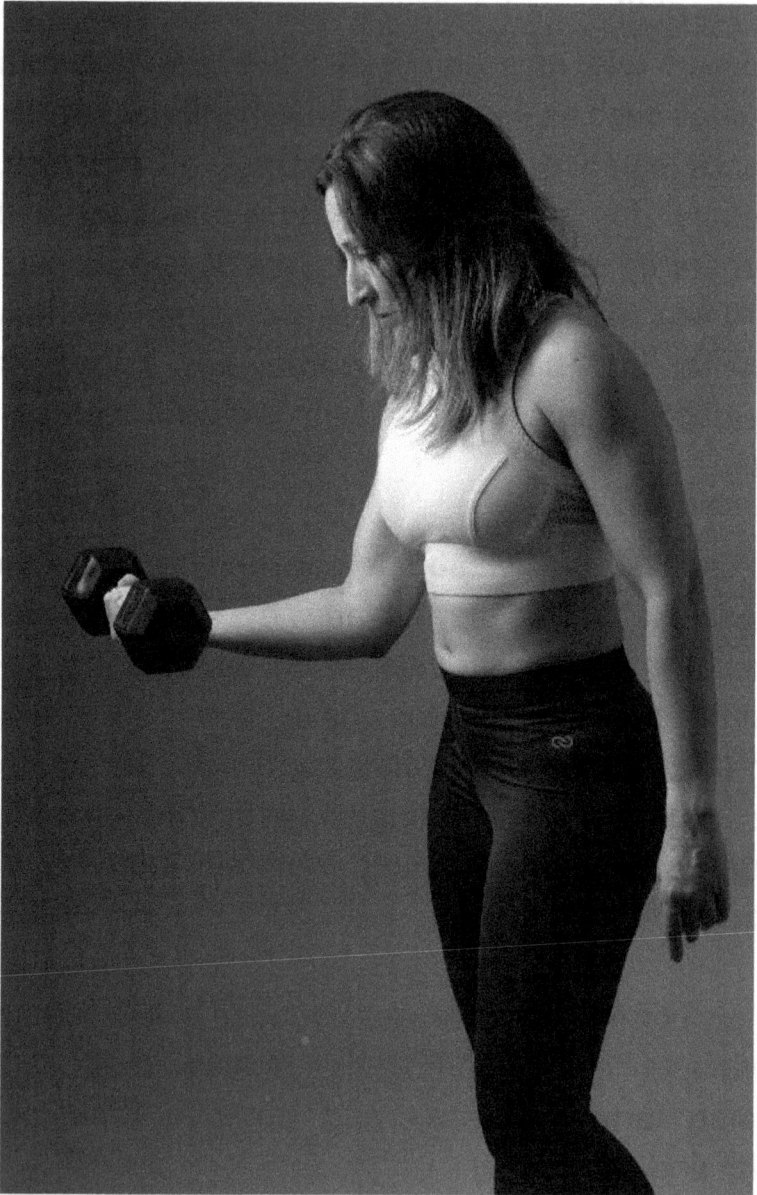

A Comprehensive Guide for Your Heart

Chapter 4

Maintaining a Healthy Weight

Understanding Body Mass Index (BMI)

Body Mass Index (BMI) is a widely used metric that helps individuals gauge their body weight in relation to their height. It is calculated by dividing a person's weight in kilograms by the square of their height in meters.

This simple formula provides a numerical value that categorizes individuals into different weight classifications: underweight, normal weight, overweight, and obese.

Understanding BMI is essential for those looking to prevent coronary artery disease, as excess body weight is a significant risk factor for heart-related issues.

A BMI below 18.5 is classified as underweight, while a BMI between 18.5 and 24.9 is considered normal weight. Individuals with a BMI ranging from 25 to 29.9 are categorized as overweight, and those with a BMI of 30 or above are classified as obese.

Each category carries its own health implications, particularly concerning cardiovascular health. Research indicates that higher BMI levels are associated with increased risks of hypertension, high cholesterol, and diabetes, all of which are contributors to coronary artery disease.

It is important to note, however, that BMI is not a definitive measure of body fat or overall health. It does not differentiate between muscle and fat, meaning that muscular individuals may fall into the overweight or obese categories despite having low body fat.

Therefore, while BMI can serve as a useful screening tool, it should be considered alongside other assessments such as waist circumference and body composition analysis for a more comprehensive understanding of one's health status.

For individuals aiming to prevent coronary artery disease, maintaining a healthy BMI is just one aspect of a holistic approach to heart health. A balanced diet rich in fruits, vegetables, whole grains, and healthy fats, combined with regular physical activity, can significantly influence body weight and overall cardiovascular health.

Monitoring BMI can help track progress and motivate individuals to adopt healthier lifestyle choices, making it a valuable component of a preventive health strategy.

In conclusion, understanding Body Mass Index is crucial for those focused on preventing coronary artery disease. While it offers a straightforward way to assess weight status, it should be interpreted with caution and used in conjunction with other health measures.

By aiming for a healthy BMI through informed lifestyle choices, individuals can take proactive steps toward reducing their risk of heart disease and enhancing their overall well-being.

Strategies for Weight Management

Weight management plays a crucial role in preventing coronary artery disease (CAD) as it directly influences heart health, blood pressure, and cholesterol levels. Effective strategies for managing weight can help reduce the risk of CAD and improve overall cardiovascular fitness.

One key approach is to adopt a balanced diet that emphasizes whole foods. Incorporating fruits, vegetables, whole grains, lean proteins, and healthy fats can create a nutrient-dense diet that supports weight loss and overall heart health. Avoiding processed foods, high-sugar snacks, and trans fats is essential, as these can contribute to unhealthy weight gain and increased cardiovascular risk.

Portion control is another vital aspect of weight management. Understanding serving sizes and practicing mindful eating can help individuals avoid overeating. When dining, it is beneficial to focus on the meal at hand, savoring each bite and listening to the body's hunger cues.

This practice helps in recognizing satiety signals, which can prevent excessive calorie intake. Keeping a food diary can also be an effective strategy, as it encourages awareness of eating habits and promotes accountability, allowing individuals to make healthier choices over time.

Regular physical activity complements dietary changes and is essential for maintaining a healthy weight. Engaging in at least 150 minutes of moderate-intensity aerobic exercise each week can significantly benefit heart health and support weight management.

Activities such as brisk walking, cycling, swimming, or dancing not only burn calories but also improve cardiovascular endurance and overall fitness. Incorporating strength training exercises at least twice a week can further enhance metabolic rate and promote muscle mass, which aids in weight loss and maintenance.

Setting realistic goals is crucial for sustainable weight management. Individuals should aim for gradual weight loss rather than drastic changes, as this approach is more likely to be maintained long-term.

Aiming for a weight loss of 1 to 2 pounds per week is a healthy target. Additionally, establishing specific, measurable, achievable, relevant, and time-bound (SMART) goals can provide clarity and motivation. By celebrating small successes along the way, individuals can maintain commitment to their weight management journey while focusing on their overall heart health.

Lastly, seeking support from healthcare professionals or weight management programs can be beneficial for those struggling to manage their weight independently. Professional guidance can provide personalized strategies tailored to individual needs, preferences, and health conditions.

Group support or counseling can also foster a sense of community, making the weight management process more enjoyable and less isolating. By integrating these strategies into daily life, individuals can significantly reduce their risk of coronary artery disease and enhance their long-term heart health.

The Impact of Weight on Heart Health

Excess weight has been identified as a significant risk factor for the development of coronary artery disease (CAD). The correlation between obesity and heart health is well-documented, with studies consistently showing that individuals with higher body mass indices (BMIs) face an increased likelihood of cardiovascular issues.

Fatty deposits can lead to inflammation and a buildup of plaque in the arteries, which narrows the passages that blood travels through, significantly elevating the risk of heart attacks and strokes.

The mechanisms by which weight influences heart health are multifaceted. Excess body fat can disrupt normal metabolic processes, leading to conditions such as insulin resistance and type 2 diabetes, both of which are closely linked to cardiovascular problems.

Additionally, obesity often leads to elevated blood pressure and dyslipidemia—characterized by increased levels of LDL cholesterol and triglycerides—further straining the heart and vascular system. These conditions create a vicious cycle; as one risk factor exacerbates another, the overall burden on heart health intensifies.

Weight loss has been shown to have a beneficial effect on cardiovascular health, even modest reductions can yield significant improvements. Research indicates that losing just 5-10% of body weight can lead to meaningful changes in blood pressure, cholesterol levels, and overall heart function.

These improvements can reduce the risk of developing CAD and enhance the effectiveness of other preventive measures, such as dietary changes and increased physical activity. Therefore, even small lifestyle adjustments can have a profound impact on heart health.

Maintaining a healthy weight is not only about avoiding heart disease but also about improving overall well-being. A balanced diet rich in fruits, vegetables, whole grains, and lean proteins, combined with regular physical activity, is essential for weight management.

These lifestyle choices contribute not only to weight loss but also to improved heart health by reducing inflammation and enhancing circulation. The integration of these habits into daily life can foster a sustained commitment to heart health.

In conclusion, the impact of weight on heart health underscores the importance of proactive measures for preventing coronary artery disease. By understanding the relationship between excess weight and cardiovascular risk, individuals can take informed steps toward achieving and maintaining a healthy weight.

This proactive approach not only helps in preventing CAD but also enhances overall quality of life, making it essential for those committed to heart health.

How To Prevent Coronary Artery Disease

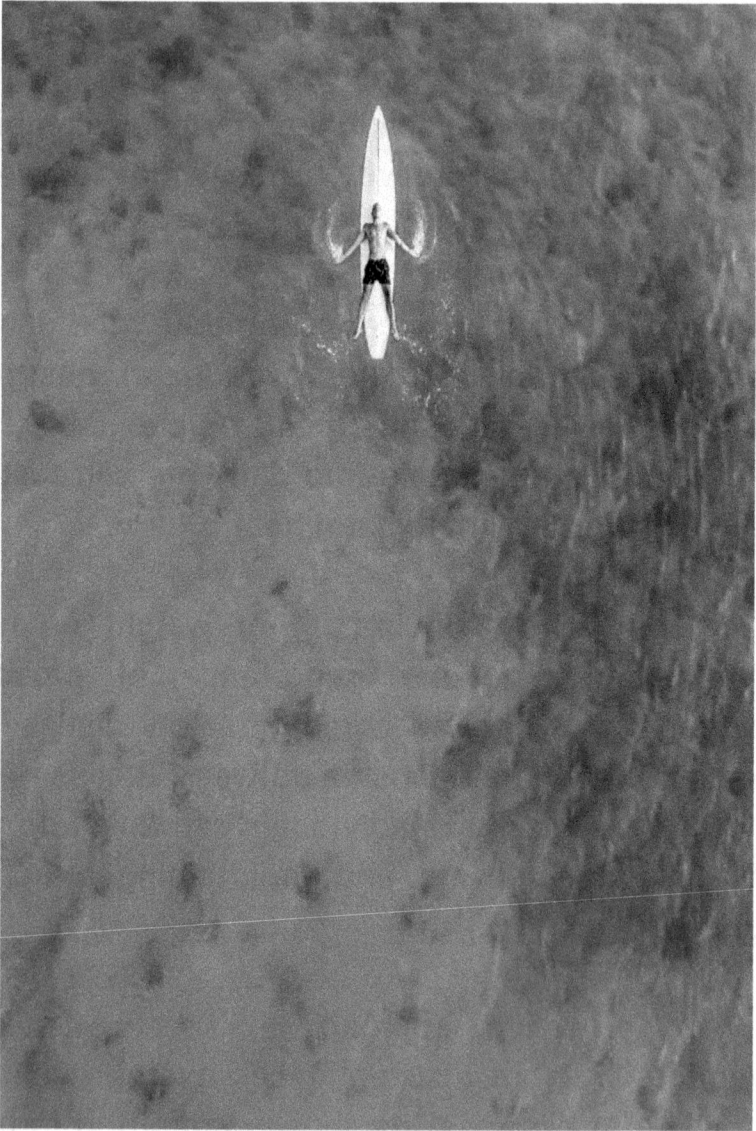

Chapter 5

Managing Stress for Heart Health

The Connection Between Stress and Heart Disease

Stress is a common experience in modern life, affecting individuals across all demographics. However, its impact on physical health is particularly significant, especially concerning heart disease. Research has established a strong correlation between chronic stress and the development of coronary artery disease (CAD).

Stress triggers a series of physiological responses in the body, including the release of stress hormones such as cortisol and adrenaline. These hormones can lead to increased heart rate and blood pressure, which over time can contribute to the hardening and narrowing of the arteries.

The mechanisms through which stress influences heart health are complex. When under stress, individuals may engage in unhealthy coping behaviors, such as smoking, overeating, or consuming alcohol. These behaviors further exacerbate the risk factors associated with CAD, including high cholesterol and obesity.

Additionally, stress can lead to inflammation in the body, a key factor in the development of cardiovascular diseases. Chronic inflammation can damage blood vessels and promote the formation of plaque in the arteries, ultimately leading to cardiovascular complications.

Moreover, stress can directly affect the heart. Studies have shown that individuals who experience high levels of stress are more likely to have elevated blood pressure and abnormal heart rhythms. This physiological strain on the heart can lead to an increased risk of heart attacks and strokes. The connection between stress and heart disease is particularly concerning for those with pre-existing conditions, as stress can exacerbate symptoms and accelerate disease progression.

Understanding this connection is crucial for individuals seeking to prevent CAD, as managing stress is an integral part of maintaining heart health.

To mitigate the effects of stress on heart health, individuals can adopt various coping strategies. Regular physical activity is one of the most effective ways to reduce stress levels while simultaneously promoting cardiovascular health.

Activities such as walking, jogging, or yoga not only help in stress relief but also improve circulation and lower blood pressure. Mindfulness practices, such as meditation and deep-breathing exercises, can also be beneficial in managing stress. These techniques promote relaxation and can help individuals develop healthier responses to stressors in their lives.

In conclusion, the relationship between stress and heart disease highlights the importance of addressing mental and emotional well-being as part of a comprehensive approach to preventing coronary artery disease.

By recognizing the signs of stress and implementing effective stress management techniques, individuals can significantly reduce their risk of developing CAD. Taking proactive steps to manage stress not only benefits heart health but also enhances overall quality of life, paving the way for a healthier future.

Stress Reduction Techniques

Stress plays a significant role in the development of coronary artery disease, as it can lead to harmful behaviors and physiological changes that increase cardiovascular risk. Understanding and implementing effective stress reduction techniques is essential for anyone looking to prevent heart disease.

These techniques not only help in managing stress but also contribute to overall heart health by promoting relaxation, improving emotional well-being, and fostering healthier lifestyle choices.

One of the most widely recognized techniques for stress reduction is mindfulness meditation. Mindfulness encourages individuals to focus on the present moment, acknowledging thoughts and feelings without judgment. Research has shown that regular mindfulness practice can lower blood pressure, reduce anxiety, and improve heart health. Simple practices such as deep breathing exercises, guided imagery, or body scanning can be incorporated into daily routines, making it accessible for anyone, regardless of their experience level.

Physical activity is another powerful tool for stress management. Engaging in regular exercise releases endorphins, the body's natural mood lifters, which can help alleviate stress and anxiety. Aerobic exercises such as walking, jogging, swimming, or cycling are particularly effective in promoting cardiovascular health.

Additionally, incorporating activities such as yoga or tai chi can provide both physical and mental benefits, combining movement with mindfulness, which enhances relaxation and reduces stress levels.

Social support is crucial in managing stress and maintaining heart health. Building strong relationships with family, friends, and community members can provide emotional assistance during challenging times.

Activities such as joining a support group, participating in social clubs, or simply spending quality time with loved ones can strengthen these connections. Sharing experiences and feelings with others who understand the challenges of preventing coronary artery disease can also foster a sense of belonging and reduce feelings of isolation.

Lastly, adopting a balanced lifestyle that includes adequate sleep, healthy nutrition, and time for relaxation is vital for stress reduction. Sleep deprivation can exacerbate stress and negatively impact heart health. Prioritizing sleep hygiene, such as maintaining a consistent sleep schedule and creating a restful environment, can enhance overall well-being.

Furthermore, a nutritious diet rich in fruits, vegetables, whole grains, and healthy fats not only supports heart health but also helps stabilize mood and reduce stress levels, creating a holistic approach to preventing coronary artery disease.

Mindfulness and Relaxation Practices

Mindfulness and relaxation practices play a critical role in preventing coronary artery disease (CAD) by reducing stress and promoting overall heart health. Chronic stress is a significant risk factor for CAD, as it can lead to unhealthy behaviors such as poor diet, lack of exercise, and smoking.

Engaging in mindfulness and relaxation techniques can help individuals manage their stress levels, thereby reducing their risk of developing heart-related issues. By incorporating these practices into daily routines, individuals can foster a greater sense of well-being and resilience against the pressures of life.

Mindfulness involves being fully present in the moment and aware of one's thoughts, feelings, and surroundings without judgment. This practice can be cultivated through various techniques such as meditation, deep breathing exercises, and mindful walking.

Research has shown that mindfulness can lower blood pressure, improve heart rate variability, and reduce the production of stress hormones, all of which contribute to better cardiovascular health. Regular mindfulness practice can also enhance emotional regulation, leading to healthier coping mechanisms in response to stress.

Relaxation techniques, including progressive muscle relaxation, guided imagery, and gentle yoga, can further support heart health by lowering physiological stress responses. Progressive muscle relaxation involves tensing and then relaxing different muscle groups, promoting physical relaxation and reducing tension. Guided imagery uses visualization to create a calming mental space, which can help decrease anxiety and improve mood.

Gentle yoga combines physical movement with breath awareness, promoting relaxation and flexibility while also enhancing cardiovascular function. Incorporating these techniques into daily life can lead to significant improvements in both mental and physical health.

The benefits of mindfulness and relaxation extend beyond immediate stress relief. Studies suggest that individuals who regularly practice these techniques have lower levels of inflammation and improved endothelial function, both of which are vital for maintaining heart health.

Additionally, these practices can encourage healthier lifestyle choices, such as increased physical activity and a balanced diet, which are essential components of CAD prevention. By fostering a mindful approach to life, individuals are more likely to prioritize their health and make decisions that support their cardiovascular well-being.

To effectively integrate mindfulness and relaxation practices into your daily routine, start by setting aside a few minutes each day for dedicated practice. This could be as simple as a short meditation session, a few minutes of deep breathing, or a gentle yoga class.

As you become more comfortable with these techniques, gradually increase the duration and frequency of your practice. Consider joining a local class or using online resources to stay motivated and learn new methods. By making mindfulness and relaxation a priority, you can significantly reduce your risk of coronary artery disease and enhance your overall quality of life.

How To Prevent Coronary Artery Disease

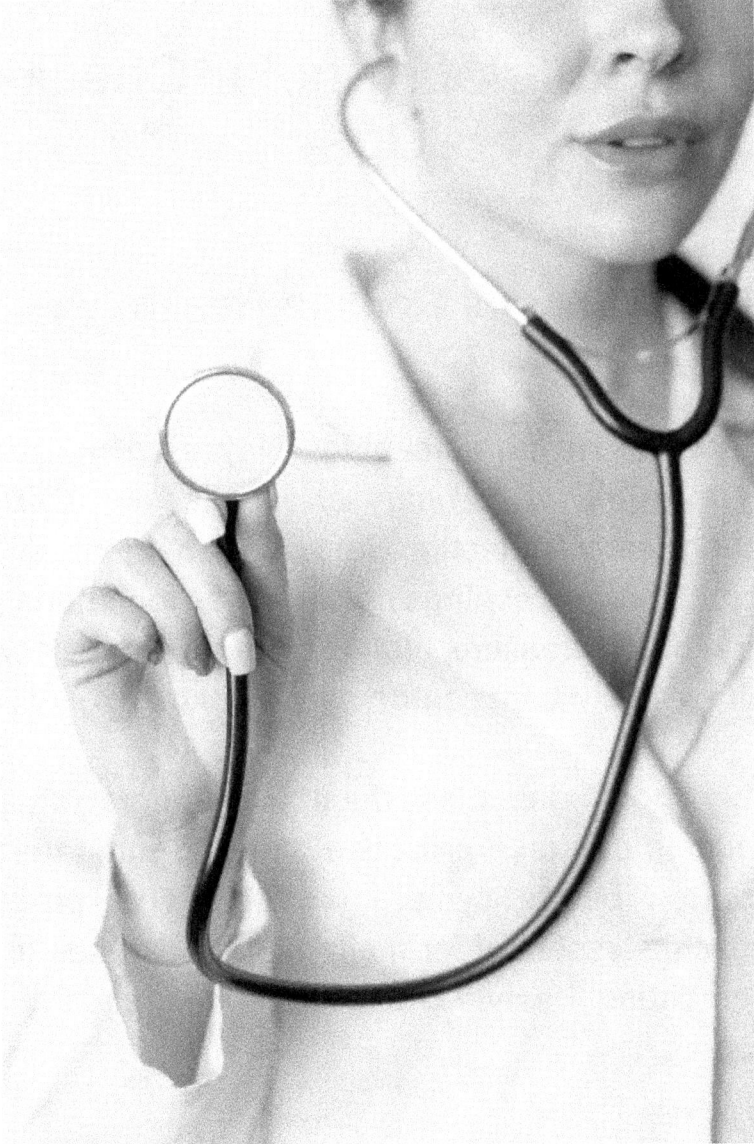

A Comprehensive Guide for Your Heart

Chapter 6

The Role of Regular Check-Ups

Importance of Routine Health Screenings

Routine health screenings play a crucial role in the prevention of coronary artery disease (CAD) by enabling early detection and management of risk factors. These screenings help identify conditions such as high blood pressure, high cholesterol, and diabetes, which are significant contributors to CAD.

By monitoring these health indicators regularly, individuals can take proactive steps to mitigate their risk, often before symptoms arise. This proactive approach is essential for maintaining heart health and implementing lifestyle changes that can lead to better outcomes.

One of the primary benefits of routine health screenings is that they provide a comprehensive overview of an individual's cardiovascular health. Screenings typically include blood tests, blood pressure measurements, and assessments of body mass index (BMI).

These evaluations offer insight into how lifestyle choices, such as diet and exercise, affect heart health. For instance, elevated cholesterol levels can prompt discussions about dietary modifications and physical activity, empowering individuals to make informed decisions that support their heart health.

In addition to identifying existing health issues, routine screenings can also serve as a motivational tool. When individuals see measurable results from their health assessments, they may feel more inclined to adopt healthier habits. For example, understanding the impact of weight loss on blood pressure or cholesterol levels can encourage sustained efforts toward fitness and nutrition.

This connection between screening results and personal health can be a powerful catalyst for change, reinforcing the importance of regular check-ups and the proactive management of health.

Moreover, routine health screenings facilitate early intervention, which is critical in preventing the progression of coronary artery disease. If a screening reveals risk factors such as elevated blood sugar or cholesterol levels, healthcare providers can recommend specific interventions, including lifestyle changes or medication.

Early intervention not only reduces the risk of developing CAD but also decreases the chances of experiencing serious complications, such as heart attacks or strokes. By addressing these issues promptly, individuals can significantly improve their long-term health outcomes.

Finally, the importance of routine health screenings extends beyond individual health; they also contribute to community health awareness. When people prioritize their screenings, it encourages others to do the same, fostering a culture of health and prevention.

Public health campaigns often highlight the significance of regular check-ups and screenings, aiming to reduce the overall incidence of coronary artery disease within the community.

By understanding the importance of routine health screenings, individuals can take charge of their cardiovascular health and inspire others to follow suit, ultimately leading to healthier populations and reduced healthcare costs related to heart disease.

Key Tests for Heart Health

Understanding your heart health is crucial in the prevention of coronary artery disease (CAD). Various tests can provide valuable insights into your cardiovascular status, allowing you to make informed decisions about your health.

Regular screening can help identify risk factors early, enabling proactive measures to mitigate potential issues. This subchapter will explore key tests that everyone should consider as part of their heart health maintenance plan.

One of the most common tests used to assess heart health is the lipid panel. This blood test measures levels of cholesterol and triglycerides in your bloodstream. High levels of low-density lipoprotein (LDL), often referred to as "bad" cholesterol, and low levels of high-density lipoprotein (HDL), or "good" cholesterol, can significantly increase your risk of developing CAD.

By understanding your lipid levels, you can work with your healthcare provider to develop a plan to manage and optimize your cholesterol levels, which may include lifestyle changes and, if necessary, medications.

Another critical test is the blood pressure measurement. Hypertension, or high blood pressure, is a significant risk factor for CAD. Regular monitoring of your blood pressure helps identify whether you fall within a healthy range or if you need to take action to lower it.

Maintaining optimal blood pressure can be achieved through lifestyle modifications such as adopting a heart-healthy diet, engaging in regular physical activity, and managing stress. For individuals with consistently high readings, medication may also be required.

An electrocardiogram (ECG or EKG) is a non-invasive test that records the electrical activity of the heart. This test can help detect irregularities in heart rhythms and identify potential heart problems. An abnormal ECG can signal underlying conditions such as arrhythmias or ischemia, which can contribute to CAD.

Understanding these issues early on allows for timely interventions, which can include lifestyle changes or medical treatments to improve heart function and overall health.

Stress testing is another valuable assessment in evaluating heart health. This test typically involves monitoring your heart while you exercise, providing insights into how well your heart copes with physical stress.

It can reveal issues that might not be apparent at rest, such as reduced blood flow to the heart muscle. This information is crucial for individuals at risk for CAD, as it helps determine the need for further diagnostic testing or intervention.

In conclusion, regularly scheduled heart health tests are essential in the prevention of coronary artery disease. By understanding and proactively managing factors such as cholesterol levels, blood pressure, heart rhythm, and stress responses, individuals can significantly reduce their risk of developing CAD. Engaging with healthcare professionals and committing to a routine of testing and lifestyle management can lead to lasting improvements in heart health and overall well-being.

Working with Healthcare Providers

Working with healthcare providers is a crucial component in the prevention of coronary artery disease (CAD). Establishing a strong partnership with your healthcare team allows for tailored strategies that align with your individual health needs and risk factors.

This proactive collaboration can lead to better management of existing conditions and the implementation of preventive measures. Engaging in open communication with your healthcare provider helps ensure that you are informed about your health status and the necessary steps to maintain cardiovascular health.

When seeking to prevent CAD, it is essential to have regular check-ups with your healthcare provider. These visits provide an opportunity to monitor key health indicators such as blood pressure, cholesterol levels, and blood sugar.

Regular screenings can help identify any potential risk factors early on, enabling timely intervention. Your provider can also help you understand your family history and lifestyle choices that may contribute to your risk, allowing for a more personalized prevention plan.

Education plays a vital role in your partnership with healthcare providers. It is important to stay informed about coronary artery disease, its risk factors, and the latest research on prevention strategies. Your provider can offer valuable resources, including educational materials and recommendations for reputable websites or support groups.

By actively participating in your health education, you can make more informed decisions about your lifestyle and treatment options, enhancing your ability to prevent CAD effectively.

In addition to standard medical advice, healthcare providers may recommend referrals to specialists, such as dietitians or cardiologists. These professionals can offer targeted guidance in areas like nutrition, exercise, and stress management, which are all critical in reducing the risk of CAD. Collaborating with a multidisciplinary team allows for a comprehensive approach to heart health, addressing various aspects of wellness that contribute to overall cardiovascular fitness.

Finally, it is essential to advocate for yourself within the healthcare system. Do not hesitate to ask questions or express concerns about your heart health during appointments. Establishing a rapport with your provider can foster an environment where you feel comfortable discussing any symptoms, lifestyle changes, or new research you may have encountered.

By being an active participant in your healthcare journey, you empower yourself to take control of your cardiovascular health and significantly reduce the risk of developing coronary artery disease.

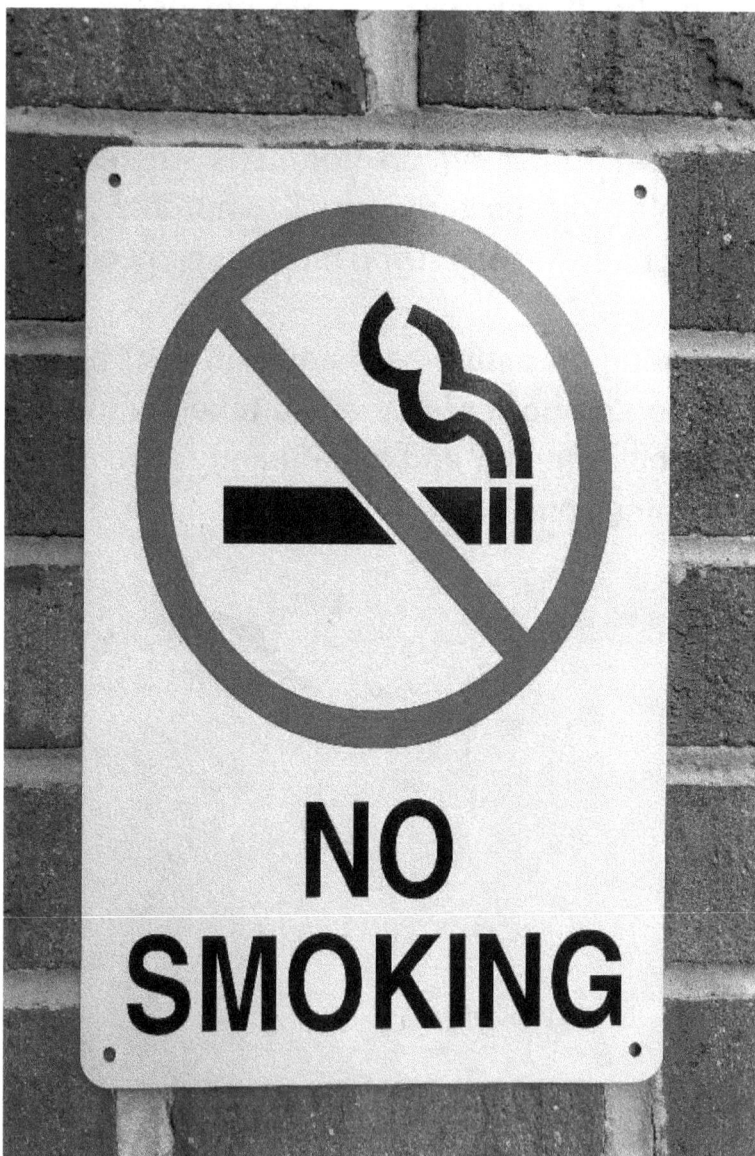

Chapter 7

Avoiding Tobacco and Limiting Alcohol

Effects of Smoking on Heart Health

Smoking has profound and detrimental effects on heart health, significantly increasing the risk of coronary artery disease (CAD). The toxic chemicals in cigarette smoke lead to the damage of blood vessels and the heart muscle itself.

Nicotine, one of the primary components of tobacco, causes an increase in heart rate and blood pressure, putting extra strain on the cardiovascular system. Over time, this heightened stress can contribute to the development of atherosclerosis, a condition characterized by the buildup of plaque in the arteries, which is a major contributor to CAD.

In addition to nicotine, smoking introduces a multitude of harmful substances into the bloodstream, including carbon monoxide and tar. Carbon monoxide reduces the amount of oxygen that can be carried by red blood cells, forcing the heart to work harder to supply the body with adequate oxygen.

This increased workload can lead to an enlarged heart and eventually heart failure. Tar, on the other hand, causes inflammation and damage to lung tissue, which can further exacerbate cardiovascular problems by reducing overall oxygen levels and leading to a cycle of poor heart health.

The effects of smoking on blood pressure and cholesterol levels are equally concerning. Smokers are more likely to have elevated levels of low-density lipoprotein (LDL) cholesterol, often referred to as "bad" cholesterol, while simultaneously having lower levels of high-density lipoprotein (HDL) cholesterol, known as "good" cholesterol. This imbalance further promotes the development of arterial plaque.

Additionally, smoking contributes to increased blood pressure, as the chemicals in cigarettes cause blood vessels to narrow, limiting blood flow and increasing the risk of blood clots, which can lead to heart attacks.

Quitting smoking is one of the most effective steps individuals can take to improve their heart health and reduce the risk of coronary artery disease. Research indicates that within just a few weeks of quitting, heart rate and blood pressure begin to stabilize, and within a year, the risk of heart disease is significantly reduced.

The circulation improves, and the lungs show signs of recovery, contributing to better overall cardiovascular health. Support systems, including counseling and nicotine replacement therapies, can greatly aid individuals in their journey to quit smoking.

Preventing coronary artery disease requires a multifaceted approach, with smoking cessation being a critical component. By understanding the detrimental effects of smoking on heart health, individuals can make informed decisions to protect their cardiovascular system.

Emphasizing the importance of a healthy lifestyle, including a balanced diet, regular exercise, and avoiding tobacco, can lead to significant improvements in heart health and a reduced risk of developing coronary artery disease.

Benefits of Quitting Smoking

Quitting smoking is one of the most significant steps individuals can take to prevent coronary artery disease. The harmful effects of tobacco on the cardiovascular system are well-documented, with smoking being a major risk factor for heart disease. When a person stops smoking, their body begins to heal almost immediately.

Within just 20 minutes, heart rate and blood pressure drop, leading to improved cardiac function. Over time, the risk of heart disease decreases significantly, making quitting an essential goal for anyone concerned about their heart health.

How To Prevent Coronary Artery Disease

One of the key benefits of quitting smoking is the reduction of harmful substances in the body. Cigarette smoke contains thousands of chemicals, many of which are toxic and can lead to systemic inflammation and arterial damage. When an individual stops smoking, the body starts to clear these toxins, which can lead to improved blood flow and reduced plaque buildup in the arteries.

This process not only enhances cardiovascular health but also lowers the chances of developing other related conditions, such as stroke and peripheral artery disease.

Moreover, quitting smoking improves overall respiratory health, which is closely tied to cardiovascular fitness. Smokers often experience reduced lung function and chronic respiratory issues, hindering their ability to engage in physical activity. Once a person quits, lung function begins to improve, making exercise more accessible and enjoyable. Regular physical activity is crucial for maintaining heart health, as it strengthens the heart muscle, improves circulation, and helps manage weight, all of which are vital in preventing coronary artery disease.

In addition to physical health benefits, there are psychological advantages associated with quitting smoking. Many individuals report increased mental clarity and improved mood after they stop smoking. The reduction in anxiety and stress related to nicotine dependence can lead to a more positive outlook on life. Furthermore, the act of quitting can enhance self-esteem and a sense of accomplishment, which can motivate individuals to adopt other healthy behaviors, such as better nutrition and regular exercise, further contributing to heart disease prevention.

Finally, quitting smoking can have significant financial benefits. The cost of purchasing cigarettes adds up quickly, and by eliminating this expense, individuals can redirect their finances towards healthier lifestyle choices. Investing in nutritious foods, gym memberships, or even heart health screenings can make a substantial difference in overall well-being.

In summary, quitting smoking not only provides immediate and long-term health benefits related to the prevention of coronary artery disease but also fosters a healthier, more fulfilling lifestyle.

Alcohol Consumption Guidelines

Alcohol consumption guidelines play a crucial role in maintaining heart health, particularly for individuals looking to prevent coronary artery disease (CAD). While some research suggests that moderate alcohol consumption may have cardiovascular benefits, it is essential to approach this topic with caution.

Understanding the distinction between moderate and excessive drinking is vital, as the latter can lead to various health issues, including hypertension, obesity, and liver disease, all of which are risk factors for CAD.

Moderate alcohol consumption is generally defined as up to one drink per day for women and up to two drinks per day for men. This guideline is based on studies indicating that light to moderate drinking may be associated with a lower risk of heart disease. The potential benefits are thought to arise from the effects of alcohol on raising high-density lipoprotein (HDL) cholesterol levels and improving insulin sensitivity.

However, it is important to note that these benefits can be achieved through other means, such as a balanced diet and regular exercise, making alcohol consumption unnecessary for heart health.

Individuals with a history of heart disease, high blood pressure, diabetes, or addiction issues should consult their healthcare providers before consuming alcohol. For these individuals, even moderate drinking might pose significant risks.

Additionally, certain medications used to manage heart conditions can interact negatively with alcohol, leading to dangerous side effects. Therefore, personal health history and current medical conditions are critical factors to consider when evaluating the role of alcohol in one's lifestyle.

For those who choose to consume alcohol, it is essential to do so mindfully and in moderation. This means being aware of the types of beverages consumed, as some options can be higher in sugar and calories, which may contribute to weight gain and increased heart disease risk.

Opting for lower-calorie drinks, like wine or light beer, and incorporating alcohol-free days into the week can help mitigate potential adverse effects while enjoying social occasions.

Ultimately, the decision to consume alcohol should be made with a clear understanding of its implications for heart health. While moderate drinking may fit into a heart-healthy lifestyle for some, it is not a requirement for preventing coronary artery disease.

Focusing on a balanced diet, regular physical activity, and maintaining a healthy weight are the most effective strategies for reducing the risk of CAD. Individuals should prioritize these factors and approach alcohol consumption with caution, ensuring that it does not detract from their overall health objectives.

How To Prevent Coronary Artery Disease

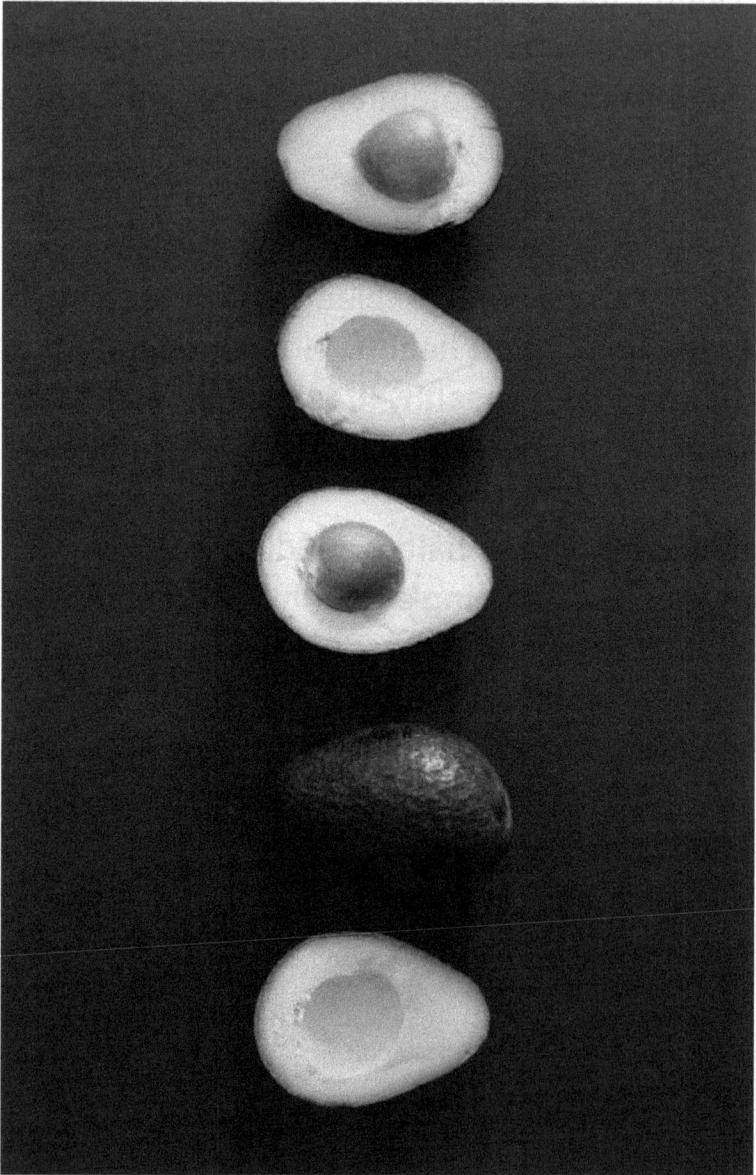

Chapter 8

Understanding and Managing Cholesterol

Types of Cholesterol

Cholesterol is a waxy substance found in every cell of the body and plays a crucial role in the production of hormones, vitamin D, and bile acids that help digest fat. However, not all cholesterol is created equal.

There are two main types of cholesterol that are significant in the context of heart health: low-density lipoprotein (LDL) and high-density lipoprotein (HDL). Understanding the differences between these types is essential for anyone looking to prevent coronary artery disease.

Low-density lipoprotein, often referred to as "bad" cholesterol, is responsible for transporting cholesterol from the liver to other parts of the body.

While some levels of LDL are necessary for bodily functions, high levels can lead to a buildup of cholesterol in the arteries. This accumulation can narrow the arteries, reducing blood flow and increasing the risk of heart attacks and strokes. Therefore, maintaining a low level of LDL cholesterol is vital for heart health and the prevention of coronary artery disease.

High-density lipoprotein, commonly known as "good" cholesterol, serves a protective role in the body. HDL helps transport cholesterol away from the arteries and back to the liver, where it can be processed and eliminated.

Higher levels of HDL cholesterol are associated with a reduced risk of heart disease, as it aids in the removal of excess cholesterol from the bloodstream. Encouraging the increase of HDL levels through lifestyle changes is an important strategy for preventing coronary artery disease.

Another type of cholesterol, known as very low-density lipoprotein (VLDL), is also important to consider. VLDL carries triglycerides, a type of fat, in the blood. Like LDL, elevated levels of VLDL can contribute to the buildup of plaque in the arteries. This makes it another risk factor for coronary artery disease. Managing triglyceride levels is crucial, and this can often be achieved through a healthy diet and regular exercise.

Finally, it is important to note that total cholesterol levels are a combination of LDL, HDL, and VLDL. While focusing on reducing LDL levels is essential, it is equally important to increase HDL levels and manage triglycerides to achieve an overall healthy cholesterol profile. Regular screening of cholesterol levels and understanding the types of cholesterol can empower individuals to take proactive steps in their heart disease prevention journey.

By making informed lifestyle choices, such as maintaining a balanced diet and engaging in regular physical activity, individuals can significantly reduce their risk of developing coronary artery disease.

How to Lower Bad Cholesterol

Lowering bad cholesterol, or low-density lipoprotein (LDL), is essential for preventing coronary artery disease. High levels of LDL can lead to plaque buildup in the arteries, which narrows them and restricts blood flow to the heart. By adopting certain lifestyle changes and dietary modifications, individuals can effectively lower their LDL cholesterol levels, thereby reducing their risk of heart disease.

One of the most significant steps in lowering bad cholesterol is improving dietary choices. Incorporating more soluble fiber into the diet can be particularly beneficial as it helps to reduce the absorption of cholesterol in the bloodstream. Foods rich in soluble fiber include oats, beans, lentils, fruits, and vegetables.

Additionally, replacing saturated fats found in red meats and full-fat dairy products with healthier fats can have a positive impact. Opting for lean meats, low-fat dairy, and incorporating sources of unsaturated fats, such as olive oil, nuts, and avocados, can help to lower LDL levels.

Regular physical activity is another effective strategy for managing cholesterol levels. Engaging in aerobic exercises, such as walking, running, swimming, or cycling, for at least 150 minutes each week can raise high-density lipoprotein (HDL) cholesterol, known as the "good" cholesterol. HDL helps to remove LDL from the bloodstream, thus contributing to a healthier cholesterol balance.

Furthermore, maintaining a healthy weight through exercise can further enhance the body's ability to manage cholesterol levels.

Quitting smoking and moderating alcohol intake are also crucial factors in lowering bad cholesterol. Smoking cessation not only improves overall heart health but also enhances HDL cholesterol levels. Moreover, excessive alcohol consumption can lead to increased cholesterol levels and should be limited to moderate amounts, which is generally defined as one drink per day for women and two drinks per day for men. Making these lifestyle adjustments can significantly contribute to better cholesterol management.

Finally, individuals should consider regular health screenings to monitor cholesterol levels and seek professional advice when needed. Consulting with healthcare providers can help tailor a cholesterol-lowering strategy that fits individual health needs and lifestyle. In some cases, medication may be necessary to manage cholesterol levels effectively. By combining lifestyle changes with medical guidance, individuals can take proactive steps to lower bad cholesterol and reduce their risk of developing coronary artery disease.

The Role of Medications

Medications play a crucial role in the prevention and management of coronary artery disease (CAD). For individuals at risk of developing CAD, understanding how these medications work can be instrumental in making informed decisions about their health. Generally, medications are used to lower cholesterol levels, manage blood pressure, and prevent blood clots. Each of these functions contributes to reducing the risk of heart attacks and other cardiovascular events, which are common complications of CAD.

Statins are one of the most frequently prescribed classes of medications for managing cholesterol levels. They work by inhibiting an enzyme involved in the production of cholesterol in the liver, effectively lowering low-density lipoprotein (LDL) cholesterol, often referred to as "bad" cholesterol.

By maintaining lower LDL levels, statins can significantly reduce the risk of plaque buildup in the arteries, which is a primary factor in the development of coronary artery disease. For individuals with elevated cholesterol levels or a family history of heart disease, statins can be a pivotal part of a comprehensive prevention strategy.

In addition to statins, other lipid-lowering agents, such as ezetimibe and PCSK9 inhibitors, may be utilized in conjunction with lifestyle changes. Ezetimibe works by reducing the amount of cholesterol absorbed from the diet, while PCSK9 inhibitors are a newer class of medications that can dramatically lower LDL levels by enhancing the liver's ability to remove cholesterol from the bloodstream.

These options are particularly useful for patients who are statin-intolerant or those who require additional lipid control beyond what statins can provide. Understanding these alternatives allows patients to work closely with their healthcare providers to tailor a medication regimen that suits their specific needs.

Blood pressure management is another critical component in preventing CAD, as hypertension can damage arteries over time and lead to heart disease. Medications such as ACE inhibitors, angiotensin II receptor blockers (ARBs), and diuretics are commonly prescribed to help manage high blood pressure.

These medications serve to relax blood vessels, reduce fluid retention, and lower overall blood pressure, thus decreasing the workload on the heart. Regular monitoring and adjustments may be necessary to ensure optimal blood pressure control, and lifestyle modifications such as diet and exercise should accompany any pharmacological interventions.

Antiplatelet medications, such as aspirin, also play a vital role in preventing coronary artery disease. These medications help prevent blood clots from forming by inhibiting the aggregation of platelets in the bloodstream. For individuals at high risk of cardiovascular events, the use of antiplatelet therapy can significantly reduce the likelihood of heart attacks or strokes. It is essential for patients to consult with their healthcare providers to determine the appropriateness of these medications based on their individual risk factors and medical history.

In conclusion, the role of medications in preventing coronary artery disease is multifaceted and should be approached as part of a comprehensive strategy that includes lifestyle modifications. Collaborating with healthcare professionals to identify the most suitable medications can empower individuals to take proactive steps in managing their heart health.

By understanding the various classes of medications available, their mechanisms, and their benefits, patients can enhance their efforts to prevent coronary artery disease and maintain a healthier heart.

How To Prevent Coronary Artery Disease

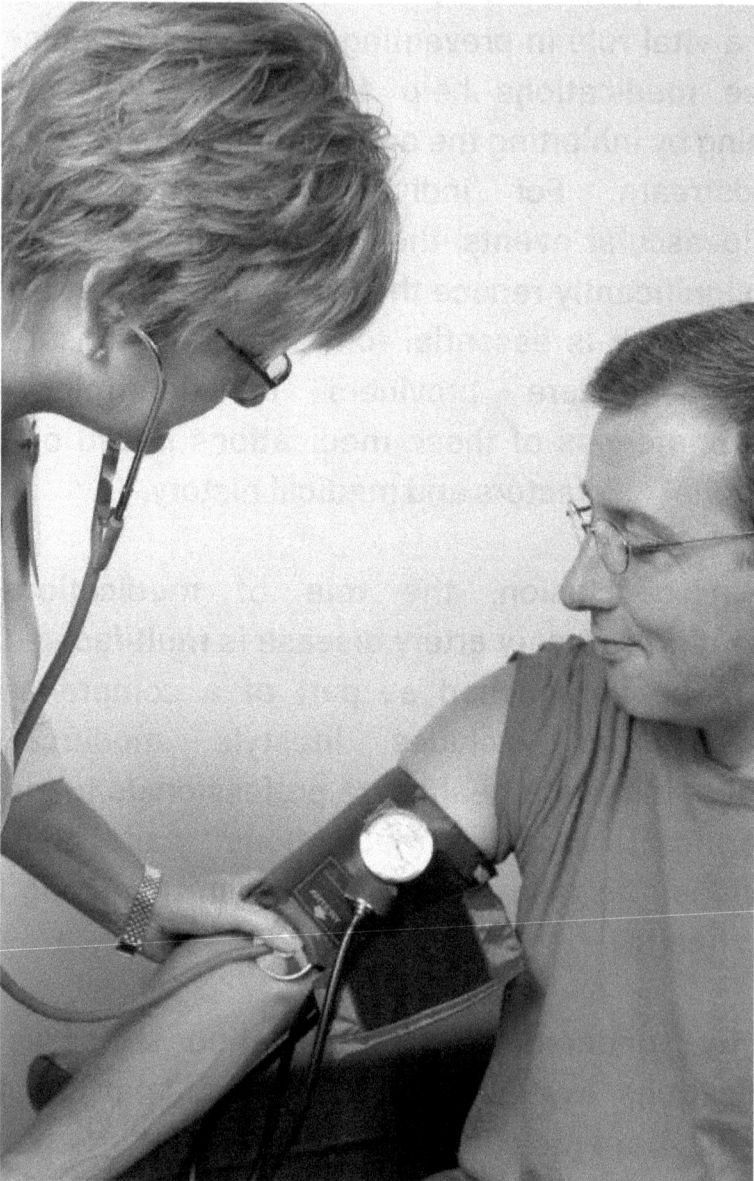

Chapter 9

Blood Pressure Management

Understanding Blood Pressure Readings

Blood pressure readings are crucial in understanding cardiovascular health and preventing coronary artery disease. These readings consist of two numbers: systolic and diastolic pressure, measured in millimeters of mercury (mmHg). Systolic pressure, the first number, indicates the pressure in the arteries when the heart beats and pumps blood.

The second number, diastolic pressure, reflects the pressure in the arteries between heartbeats when the heart is at rest. A typical blood pressure reading is expressed as systolic over diastolic, such as 120/80 mmHg, which is considered normal.

To evaluate blood pressure, it is essential to know the categories established by health organizations. Normal blood pressure is generally defined as less than 120/80 mmHg. Elevated blood pressure ranges from 120-129 systolic and less than 80 diastolic, while hypertension is classified into stages.

Stage 1 hypertension is 130-139 systolic or 80-89 diastolic, and Stage 2 hypertension is 140 or higher systolic or 90 or higher diastolic. Understanding these categories helps individuals recognize their blood pressure status and the potential risks associated with elevated readings.

Regular monitoring of blood pressure is vital for early detection of potential issues. Individuals can measure their blood pressure at home using a digital blood pressure monitor or at a healthcare provider's office. Home monitoring allows for a more comfortable and less stressful environment, which can lead to more accurate readings. Keeping a log of blood pressure readings can help identify trends and provide valuable information to healthcare professionals for risk assessment and management.

Lifestyle factors play a significant role in maintaining healthy blood pressure levels. A balanced diet rich in fruits, vegetables, whole grains, and lean proteins while low in sodium can significantly impact blood pressure regulation. Regular physical activity, aimed at achieving at least 150 minutes of moderate-intensity exercise weekly, can also help lower blood pressure and improve overall heart health.

Additionally, managing stress through mindfulness practices, adequate sleep, and avoiding tobacco and excessive alcohol consumption contributes to maintaining healthy blood pressure levels.

Understanding blood pressure readings is essential for individuals aiming to prevent coronary artery disease. By recognizing the significance of systolic and diastolic values, monitoring these readings regularly, and implementing lifestyle changes to promote cardiovascular health, individuals can take proactive steps in reducing their risk.

Consultation with healthcare professionals for personalized advice and interventions can further enhance efforts toward maintaining optimal blood pressure and preventing heart-related conditions.

Lifestyle Changes to Lower Blood Pressure

Lifestyle changes play a crucial role in managing and lowering blood pressure, which is essential for preventing coronary artery disease. The first step towards achieving healthier blood pressure levels is adopting a balanced diet. A diet rich in fruits, vegetables, whole grains, and lean proteins can significantly impact overall cardiovascular health.

The Dietary Approaches to Stop Hypertension (DASH) diet, for example, emphasizes reducing sodium intake while increasing potassium-rich foods, which can help lower blood pressure. Incorporating foods high in omega-3 fatty acids, such as salmon and walnuts, also supports heart health and can contribute to better blood pressure regulation.

Regular physical activity is another vital component of a heart-healthy lifestyle. Engaging in moderate aerobic exercise for at least 150 minutes each week can help lower blood pressure and improve overall cardiovascular fitness. Activities such as walking, swimming, and cycling not only promote heart health but also aid in weight management.

Maintaining a healthy weight is important, as excess body weight can increase blood pressure. Therefore, combining exercise with dietary changes can lead to significant improvements in blood pressure levels and overall well-being.

Stress management techniques are equally important for maintaining healthy blood pressure. Chronic stress can lead to unhealthy coping mechanisms, such as overeating or excessive alcohol consumption, both of which can contribute to high blood pressure. Techniques such as mindfulness, meditation, yoga, and deep breathing exercises can help reduce stress levels. Establishing a regular routine that includes time for relaxation and self-care can also enhance emotional well-being and mitigate the effects of stress on blood pressure.

How To Prevent Coronary Artery Disease

Limiting alcohol and avoiding tobacco products are essential lifestyle modifications for blood pressure management. Excessive alcohol consumption can raise blood pressure and contribute to weight gain, while smoking damages blood vessels and increases the risk of coronary artery disease.

If you choose to drink alcohol, moderation is key—generally defined as up to one drink per day for women and up to two drinks per day for men. Quitting smoking can have immediate and long-term benefits for heart health, and various resources are available to assist individuals in this endeavor.

Finally, regular monitoring of blood pressure is crucial for those aiming to prevent coronary artery disease. Keeping track of blood pressure readings can help individuals stay informed about their health and recognize any changes that may require attention. Collaborating with healthcare providers to develop a personalized plan that includes lifestyle changes, medication if necessary, and regular check-ups will further support blood pressure management.

By implementing these lifestyle changes, individuals can take proactive steps towards lowering their blood pressure and reducing their risk of developing coronary artery disease.

Medications for Hypertension

Medications for hypertension play a crucial role in managing blood pressure effectively, thereby reducing the risk of coronary artery disease (CAD). Hypertension, or high blood pressure, is a significant risk factor for CAD, as it can lead to damage of the heart and blood vessels over time.

By controlling blood pressure through medication, individuals can significantly decrease their chances of developing heart-related complications. It is essential to understand the various classes of medications available, their mechanisms of action, potential side effects, and the importance of adherence to prescribed treatment.

There are several classes of antihypertensive medications, including diuretics, beta-blockers, ACE inhibitors, angiotensin II receptor blockers (ARBs), calcium channel blockers, and others. Diuretics help the body eliminate excess sodium and water, reducing blood volume and lowering blood pressure. Beta-blockers work by slowing down the heart rate and reducing the force of heart contractions.

ACE inhibitors and ARBs relax blood vessels, making it easier for the heart to pump blood. Calcium channel blockers prevent calcium from entering heart and blood vessel cells, leading to relaxed blood vessels and decreased heart workload. Each class has its unique benefits and is chosen based on individual health profiles and the presence of other conditions.

While these medications are effective in controlling hypertension, they may come with potential side effects that patients should be aware of. Common side effects of diuretics include increased urination and electrolyte imbalances. Beta-blockers can cause fatigue, cold extremities, and in some cases, depression. ACE inhibitors may lead to persistent cough or elevated potassium levels.

It is vital for patients to discuss any adverse effects with their healthcare provider, as adjustments in dosage or a switch to another medication may be necessary to achieve optimal results without compromising quality of life.

Adherence to prescribed hypertension medications is essential for effective management. Non-adherence can lead to uncontrolled blood pressure, increasing the risk of heart attacks, strokes, and other cardiovascular issues.

Patients are encouraged to develop strategies for remembering to take their medications, such as setting daily reminders or using pill organizers. Regular follow-ups with healthcare providers to monitor blood pressure and adjust treatment as needed can also enhance adherence and ensure that the chosen medication remains effective.

In addition to medications, lifestyle modifications such as diet, exercise, and stress management are vital components of hypertension management and CAD prevention.

A heart-healthy diet rich in fruits, vegetables, whole grains, and lean proteins, combined with regular physical activity, can complement the effects of medication. Patients should also be encouraged to limit sodium intake, avoid excessive alcohol consumption, and quit smoking.

By combining pharmacological treatment with healthy lifestyle choices, individuals can significantly lower their blood pressure and reduce the risk of coronary artery disease, ultimately leading to better overall heart health.

How To Prevent Coronary Artery Disease

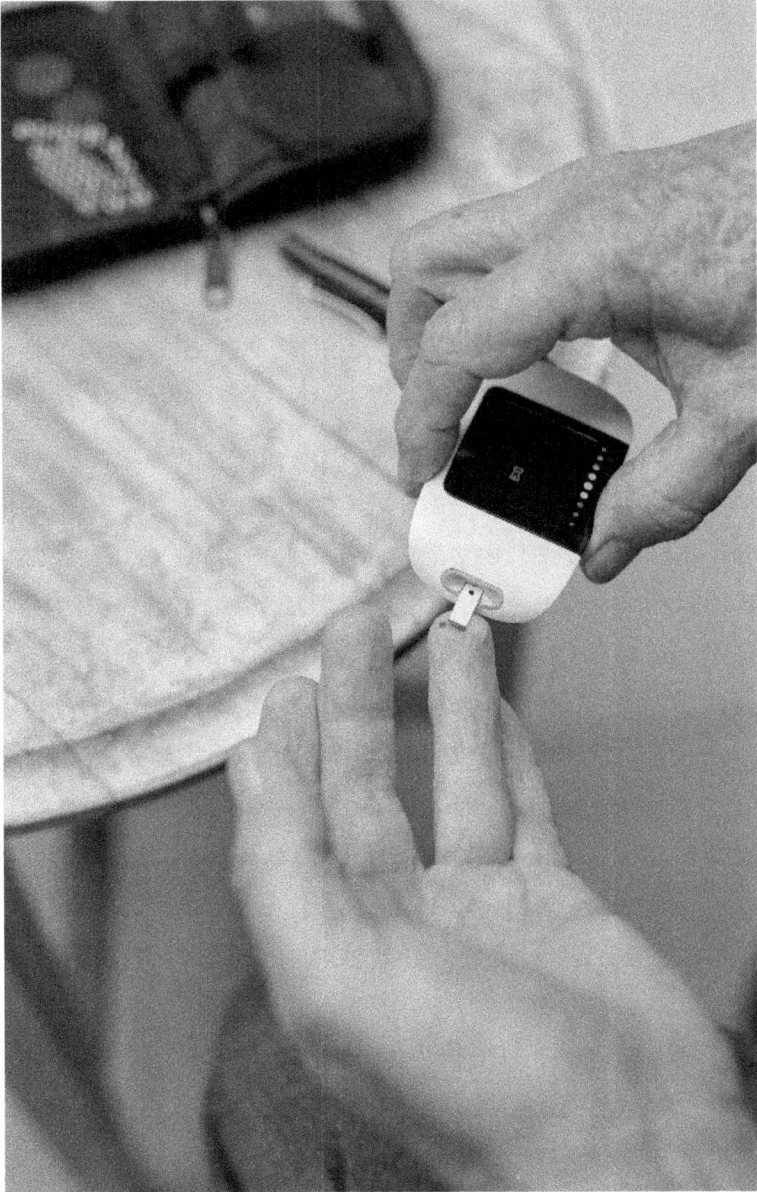

Chapter 10

The Impact of Diabetes on Heart Health

Connection Between Diabetes and Heart Disease

Diabetes and heart disease are intricately linked, forming a significant health concern for individuals at risk of coronary artery disease. People with diabetes often experience elevated blood sugar levels, which can lead to a range of complications.

Among these complications, cardiovascular disease is one of the most pressing, as diabetes alters the body's natural ability to utilize insulin and manage glucose levels, contributing to the development of atherosclerosis. This condition, characterized by the buildup of plaque in the arteries, narrows the passageways and impedes blood flow, increasing the likelihood of heart attacks and other serious cardiovascular events.

Hyperglycemia, the condition of having high blood sugar, can damage blood vessels and nerves over time. This damage affects the heart and circulation, making it crucial for individuals with diabetes to monitor their blood glucose levels closely. Research has shown that individuals with diabetes are at a higher risk of developing coronary artery disease compared to those without diabetes.

The presence of additional risk factors, such as hypertension and high cholesterol, further exacerbates this risk. Therefore, managing blood sugar levels is not only essential for diabetes control but also for maintaining heart health and preventing coronary artery disease.

Furthermore, the metabolic syndrome, a cluster of conditions that includes increased blood pressure, high blood sugar, excess body fat around the waist, and abnormal cholesterol levels, is often found in individuals with diabetes. This syndrome significantly raises the risk of heart disease, making it imperative to address all components of metabolic health.

Lifestyle interventions, such as maintaining a balanced diet, engaging in regular physical activity, and achieving a healthy weight, can be effective strategies for managing both diabetes and heart disease. These lifestyle changes not only improve glycemic control but also contribute to overall cardiovascular health.

Another important factor in the connection between diabetes and heart disease is inflammation. Chronic low-grade inflammation is common in individuals with diabetes and has been identified as a contributing factor to the development of atherosclerosis. Inflammatory markers, such as C-reactive protein, tend to be elevated in diabetic patients, which indicates an increased risk of cardiovascular events.

By adopting anti-inflammatory diets rich in omega-3 fatty acids, antioxidants, and whole foods, individuals can potentially mitigate this risk and promote heart health.

In summary, individuals aiming to prevent coronary artery disease must recognize the profound connection between diabetes and cardiovascular health. Effective management of diabetes through lifestyle modifications, routine monitoring of blood glucose levels, and a focus on reducing inflammation can significantly lower the risk of developing heart disease. By understanding this relationship and taking proactive steps, individuals can better protect their hearts and improve their overall well-being, paving the way for a healthier future.

Managing Blood Sugar Levels

Managing blood sugar levels is a critical aspect of preventing coronary artery disease (CAD). Elevated blood sugar can lead to insulin resistance, a condition where the body's cells become less responsive to insulin, resulting in higher glucose levels in the bloodstream. Over time, this can damage blood vessels and contribute to the development of atherosclerosis, the buildup of fatty deposits in the arteries. By understanding how to manage blood sugar effectively, individuals can significantly reduce their risk of CAD.

One of the most effective ways to manage blood sugar levels is through dietary choices. Consuming a balanced diet rich in whole grains, fruits, vegetables, lean proteins, and healthy fats can help maintain steady blood sugar levels. Foods with a low glycemic index are particularly beneficial, as they result in a slower, more controlled rise in blood sugar. It is also essential to monitor carbohydrate intake, as excessive consumption can lead to spikes in blood glucose. Incorporating fiber-rich foods can enhance satiety and slow down digestion, further aiding in blood sugar management.

Regular physical activity plays a vital role in controlling blood sugar levels as well. Exercise helps the body utilize glucose more efficiently, reducing insulin resistance and promoting better blood sugar control. Engaging in a combination of aerobic exercises, such as walking or cycling, and strength training can provide significant benefits. Aim for at least 150 minutes of moderate-intensity exercise each week. Additionally, incorporating movement throughout the day, like taking short walks or using stairs, can enhance overall metabolic health.

Monitoring blood sugar levels is crucial for those at risk of CAD. Individuals should consider using a blood glucose meter to track their levels, especially if they have prediabetes or diabetes.

Regular monitoring helps identify patterns and triggers that may lead to elevated blood sugar, allowing for timely adjustments in diet or activity. Consulting with healthcare professionals can provide personalized recommendations and support for effectively managing blood sugar levels.

Finally, stress management and adequate sleep are essential components of blood sugar regulation. Chronic stress can lead to hormonal imbalances that increase blood sugar levels, while insufficient sleep can disrupt glucose metabolism. Implementing stress-reduction techniques such as mindfulness, meditation, or yoga can be beneficial.

Prioritizing sleep hygiene by maintaining a consistent sleep schedule and creating a restful environment can improve overall health and support blood sugar control. Together, these strategies contribute to a comprehensive approach to preventing coronary artery disease through effective management of blood sugar levels.

Prevention Strategies for Diabetics

Diabetes significantly increases the risk of coronary artery disease (CAD), making it crucial for diabetics to adopt effective prevention strategies. One of the most impactful approaches is to maintain optimal blood glucose levels. Regular monitoring of blood sugar is essential for assessing one's control over diabetes. Individuals should work closely with healthcare providers to establish personalized targets and develop a plan that may include dietary adjustments, medication, and lifestyle modifications.

Keeping blood glucose within the target range can reduce the long-term complications associated with diabetes, including those affecting the heart and blood vessels.

In addition to blood glucose management, a heart-healthy diet plays a vital role in preventing coronary artery disease for diabetics. A diet rich in whole grains, lean proteins, healthy fats, and an abundance of fruits and vegetables is recommended. These foods not only help manage blood sugar levels but also lower cholesterol and blood pressure, further reducing CAD risk.

It is important to limit the intake of refined carbohydrates, added sugars, and saturated fats. Meal planning and portion control can also assist in managing weight, which is another critical factor in both diabetes and heart health.

Regular physical activity is another cornerstone of prevention strategies for those with diabetes. Engaging in at least 150 minutes of moderate-intensity aerobic exercise each week can improve insulin sensitivity, support weight management, and enhance cardiovascular health. Activities such as walking, cycling, or swimming can easily be incorporated into daily routines.

Additionally, strength training exercises twice a week can further improve metabolic health and support muscle mass. It is advisable for individuals to consult with healthcare providers before starting any new exercise regimen, especially if they have existing health conditions.

Stress management is often overlooked but is essential for diabetics seeking to prevent coronary artery disease. Chronic stress can lead to elevated blood sugar levels and unhealthy coping mechanisms such as overeating or physical inactivity. Techniques such as mindfulness, yoga, and deep-breathing exercises can be beneficial in reducing stress levels.

Moreover, establishing a solid support network among family, friends, and healthcare professionals can provide emotional support and encouragement, helping individuals cope with the challenges of managing diabetes while maintaining heart health.

Finally, regular medical check-ups are critical for monitoring both diabetes and cardiovascular health. These appointments allow for ongoing assessment of risk factors such as blood pressure, cholesterol levels, and overall cardiovascular health. Diabetics should take an active role in their healthcare by asking questions, discussing concerns, and ensuring that all aspects of their health are being addressed. By adhering to these prevention strategies, diabetics can significantly reduce their risk of developing coronary artery disease and improve their overall quality of life.

How To Prevent Coronary Artery Disease

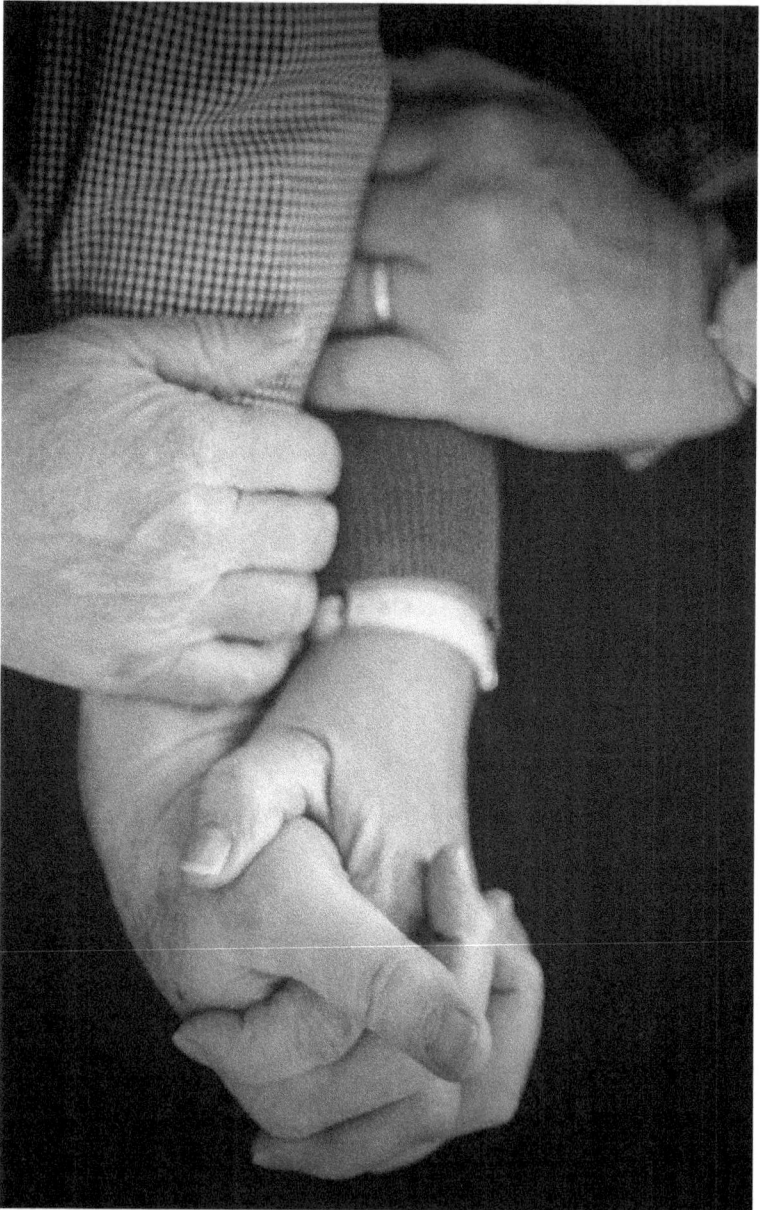

Chapter 11

Building a Support System

Importance of Social Support

Social support plays a crucial role in maintaining overall health and well-being, particularly when it comes to preventing coronary artery disease (CAD). Research consistently demonstrates that individuals with strong social networks are better equipped to manage stress, adhere to healthy lifestyle choices, and maintain positive mental health.

This support can come from family, friends, or community groups, and it often serves as a buffer against the psychological and emotional challenges that can contribute to heart disease.

One of the key benefits of social support is its impact on stress reduction. Chronic stress is a known risk factor for CAD, as it can lead to high blood pressure, increased heart rate, and unhealthy coping mechanisms such as overeating or smoking.

Individuals who feel supported by their social networks are typically more resilient in the face of stress. They are more likely to engage in protective behaviors, such as physical activity or seeking medical advice, when they have encouragement and understanding from those around them.

Moreover, social support can significantly influence health-related behaviors. People with strong social ties are often more motivated to make healthier lifestyle choices, such as maintaining a balanced diet, exercising regularly, and adhering to medical recommendations.

For example, when friends or family members participate in healthy activities together, such as cooking nutritious meals or exercising, it can create a sense of accountability and make these behaviors more enjoyable. Such collaborative efforts reinforce positive habits that are essential in preventing CAD.

In addition to promoting healthy behaviors, social support also fosters emotional well-being. Isolation and loneliness can lead to depression and anxiety, which are both associated with an increased risk of heart disease. Having a network of supportive individuals can alleviate feelings of loneliness and provide a sense of belonging.

This emotional connection can be particularly beneficial for those managing chronic conditions or facing significant lifestyle changes, as it encourages individuals to share their experiences and seek advice when needed.

Finally, the importance of social support extends beyond immediate relationships. Community involvement and belonging to support groups can provide additional resources and encouragement for individuals focused on heart health. These groups often share valuable information, strategies for lifestyle change, and emotional support, creating an environment where individuals can thrive.

By fostering connections within both personal and community settings, individuals can enhance their capacity to prevent coronary artery disease and improve their overall quality of life.

Finding Community Resources

Finding community resources is an essential step in the journey to prevent coronary artery disease. Local organizations, health departments, and non-profit groups often provide valuable information and support that can aid individuals in adopting heart-healthy lifestyles.

These resources may include educational workshops, nutritional counseling, exercise programs, and support groups tailored to those at risk for or living with heart disease. Engaging with these community offerings can empower individuals with knowledge and tools necessary for making informed health choices.

One of the first places to look for community resources is local health departments. Many health departments offer free or low-cost screenings for cardiovascular health, including blood pressure and cholesterol checks. They may also provide classes on heart health, nutrition, and physical activity.

By participating in these screenings and educational programs, individuals can gain insights into their heart health status and learn how to make lifestyle modifications to reduce risk factors associated with coronary artery disease.

Community centers and local gyms frequently host fitness classes specifically designed for those looking to improve their cardiovascular health. These classes might include aerobic exercises, yoga, or strength training, all of which can play a crucial role in maintaining a healthy heart.

Additionally, many of these centers provide access to personal trainers who can create tailored exercise plans that cater to an individual's unique health profile and fitness level. Participating in these activities not only enhances physical health but also fosters a sense of community and support among peers with similar health goals.

Support groups can also be invaluable resources for those seeking to prevent coronary artery disease. Many hospitals and community organizations offer programs where individuals can share their experiences, challenges, and successes in managing their heart health.

These groups provide a platform for emotional support, encouragement, and accountability, which can be vital in maintaining motivation for lifestyle changes. Learning from others who are on the same journey can help participants feel less isolated and more empowered in their efforts to adopt heart-healthy habits.

Finally, online resources can complement local community offerings. Websites dedicated to heart health, such as those run by the American Heart Association or other reputable organizations, often feature directories of local resources, educational materials, and forums for discussion.

Social media platforms can connect individuals with local support networks and events, expanding their reach beyond physical boundaries. By leveraging both local and online resources, individuals can create a comprehensive support system that enhances their ability to prevent coronary artery disease effectively.

Engaging Family and Friends

Engaging family and friends is a crucial component in the journey to prevent coronary artery disease. When individuals take proactive steps to improve their heart health, the support and involvement of loved ones can significantly enhance motivation and accountability.

Family and friends can play a vital role in fostering a heart-healthy environment, making lifestyle changes more enjoyable and sustainable. Their participation can transform personal health goals into collective activities, encouraging everyone involved to adopt healthier habits together.

One effective way to engage family and friends is by educating them about coronary artery disease and its risk factors. Sharing information about how lifestyle choices impact heart health can help create a shared understanding of the importance of prevention.

Hosting informational sessions or casual discussions can facilitate open conversations about dietary changes, exercise routines, and the significance of regular health screenings. The more informed everyone is, the more likely they are to support each other in making healthier choices.

Incorporating group activities focused on heart health can strengthen relationships while promoting wellness. Family outings can be centered around physical activities such as hiking, biking, or participating in community sports.

Cooking healthy meals together not only makes the process enjoyable but also allows for the exchange of nutritious recipes and ideas. These shared experiences not only foster stronger bonds but also serve as a reminder of the collective commitment to preventing coronary artery disease.

Additionally, establishing a support network can enhance individual efforts to maintain a heart-healthy lifestyle. Regular check-ins with family and friends can serve as encouragement and motivation.

Whether it's weekly phone calls, group text messages, or scheduled meet-ups, these interactions can help individuals stay accountable to their health goals. Moreover, sharing successes and challenges can provide valuable insights and reinforce the importance of perseverance in the face of obstacles.

Lastly, understanding that prevention is a lifelong journey can help frame discussions with family and friends positively. It's essential to celebrate small victories and acknowledge that setbacks may occur along the way.

By fostering an environment of understanding and support, individuals can navigate their health journeys together, creating a culture of wellness that extends beyond personal goals. Engaging loved ones not only amplifies the impact of heart-healthy habits but also builds a community committed to preventing coronary artery disease.

How To Prevent Coronary Artery Disease

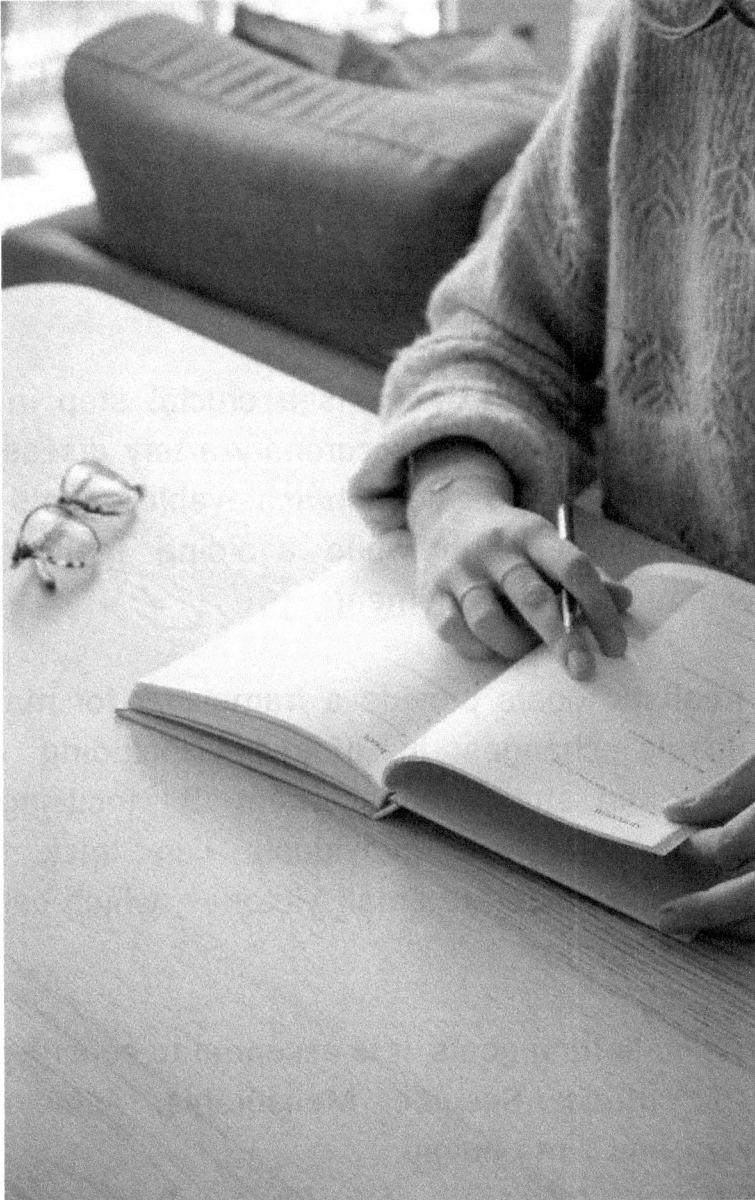

A Comprehensive Guide for Your Heart

Chapter 12

Creating a Personal Action Plan

Setting Realistic Goals

Setting realistic goals is a crucial step in the journey toward preventing coronary artery disease. It allows individuals to establish achievable targets that promote heart health while avoiding feelings of overwhelm or discouragement.

Realistic goals provide a framework for making sustainable changes in lifestyle, including diet, exercise, and stress management. By focusing on attainable objectives, individuals can track their progress and celebrate small victories, which can be highly motivating.

When setting goals, it is essential to consider the SMART criteria: Specific, Measurable, Achievable, Relevant, and Time-bound.

Specific goals outline clear and concise objectives, such as committing to a certain amount of physical activity each week. Measurable goals allow individuals to quantify their progress, such as aiming to lower cholesterol levels by a specific percentage. Achievable goals ensure that the targets set are realistic given one's current circumstances, while relevant goals align with personal health aspirations. Finally, time-bound goals provide a deadline for accountability, helping individuals stay committed to their heart health journey.

Assessing one's current lifestyle is a vital first step in goal-setting. Individuals should take an honest inventory of their eating habits, physical activity levels, stress factors, and any existing health conditions. Understanding these elements helps in establishing a baseline from which to develop realistic goals.

For instance, if someone currently engages in minimal physical activity, setting a goal to exercise for 30 minutes daily right away may be unrealistic. Instead, starting with a goal of walking for 10 minutes three times a week can build a solid foundation for gradually increasing activity levels.

In addition to individual goals, it is beneficial to set goals within a supportive network. Engaging family members or friends in the journey can create an encouraging environment that fosters accountability. Group goals, such as participating in community fitness events or cooking healthy meals together, can enhance motivation and make the process more enjoyable.

Sharing progress and challenges with others can provide valuable support and advice, further reinforcing the commitment to preventing coronary artery disease.

Finally, it is important to revisit and adjust goals as needed. Life circumstances can change, and what may have been a realistic goal at one point might no longer be attainable. Regularly evaluating goals allows individuals to adapt their plans based on progress, setbacks, or new information about heart health. This flexibility can alleviate frustration and encourage persistence, ensuring that the pursuit of a heart-healthy lifestyle remains a positive and rewarding experience.

By emphasizing realistic goal-setting, individuals can effectively work towards preventing coronary artery disease while fostering resilience and motivation along the way.

Tracking Progress

Tracking progress is a crucial aspect of preventing coronary artery disease, as it allows individuals to monitor their health and make necessary adjustments to their lifestyle. Establishing a baseline of key health indicators is the first step in this process. Individuals should regularly check their blood pressure, cholesterol levels, and blood sugar levels.

These metrics provide essential insights into heart health and help identify potential risk factors. Keeping a health journal or using mobile health applications can simplify the process of logging these measurements and tracking changes over time.

Regular physical activity is a critical component of heart health, and tracking exercise can significantly impact one's ability to prevent coronary artery disease. Setting specific fitness goals, such as walking a certain number of steps each day or engaging in cardiovascular exercises several times a week, can motivate individuals to stay active.

Wearable technology, such as fitness trackers or smartwatches, can assist in monitoring daily activity levels, heart rate, and calorie expenditure. By reviewing this data regularly, individuals can see their progress, identify patterns, and make informed decisions about their exercise routines.

Nutrition plays a vital role in heart health, and tracking dietary habits can help individuals make healthier food choices. Keeping a food diary allows individuals to record their daily intake, helping them identify areas for improvement. This practice can spotlight excessive consumption of saturated fats, sodium, and added sugars, which are linked to an increased risk of coronary artery disease.

Additionally, incorporating a variety of fruits, vegetables, whole grains, and lean proteins can be tracked to ensure a balanced diet. By monitoring dietary intake, individuals can reinforce positive habits and make informed adjustments to promote heart health.

Stress management is another critical factor in preventing coronary artery disease, and recognizing stress levels is essential for tracking progress. Individuals can benefit from mindfulness practices, such as meditation or yoga, to help manage stress effectively.

Keeping a stress journal can also be beneficial, allowing individuals to note triggers and responses to stress over time. By evaluating their emotional and psychological well-being, individuals can implement coping strategies and recognize when to seek professional help, thereby improving their overall heart health.

Finally, regular medical check-ups are essential for tracking progress in preventing coronary artery disease. Healthcare professionals can provide valuable insights based on various health metrics and risk factors, facilitating early intervention when necessary.

Engaging in open discussions with healthcare providers about personal health goals enables individuals to stay informed and accountable. By combining self-monitoring with professional guidance, individuals can create a comprehensive approach to tracking their heart health and making strides towards preventing coronary artery disease.

Staying Motivated for Long-Term Success

Staying motivated for long-term success in preventing coronary artery disease is crucial for maintaining a healthy lifestyle. The journey towards heart health is often a long and challenging one, requiring consistent effort and dedication. It is essential to establish clear, attainable goals that align with your health objectives.

These goals should focus not only on weight management and physical activity but also on maintaining a balanced diet rich in heart-healthy foods. Regularly revisiting and adjusting these goals can help keep your motivation levels high.

One effective strategy for sustaining motivation is to track your progress. Keeping a journal or using a mobile app to log dietary choices, physical activity, and health markers can provide tangible evidence of your improvements over time. This tracking allows you to celebrate small victories, which can significantly boost your morale. Additionally, sharing your journey with friends, family, or support groups can create a community of encouragement and accountability, making it easier to stay committed to your health goals.

Incorporating variety into your routine can also enhance motivation. Engaging in different types of physical activity not only prevents boredom but can also lead to discovering new interests. Whether it's trying a new workout class, hiking, swimming, or even dancing, the key is to find enjoyable activities that contribute to cardiovascular fitness.

Similarly, exploring new recipes or meal options can make healthy eating more exciting and less of a chore. This variety can help you remain engaged in your health journey.

Mindset plays a significant role in sustaining motivation. Adopting a positive attitude towards your health can help you overcome challenges and setbacks. Practicing mindfulness and self-compassion allows you to view obstacles as opportunities for growth rather than failures.

Focusing on the benefits of a heart-healthy lifestyle, such as increased energy, improved mood, and enhanced overall well-being, can reinforce your commitment to long-term success. Visualizing your future self enjoying a healthier life can serve as a powerful motivator.

Lastly, recognizing the importance of patience is vital for sustaining motivation over time. Preventing coronary artery disease is not an overnight process; it requires ongoing effort and lifestyle changes. Understand that progress may be slow and that occasional setbacks are a normal part of the journey.

By adopting a long-term perspective and celebrating gradual improvements, you can maintain your motivation and stay focused on your goal of heart health. Emphasizing the journey rather than solely the end result will help you remain committed to your health and well-being for years to come.

How To Prevent Coronary Artery Disease

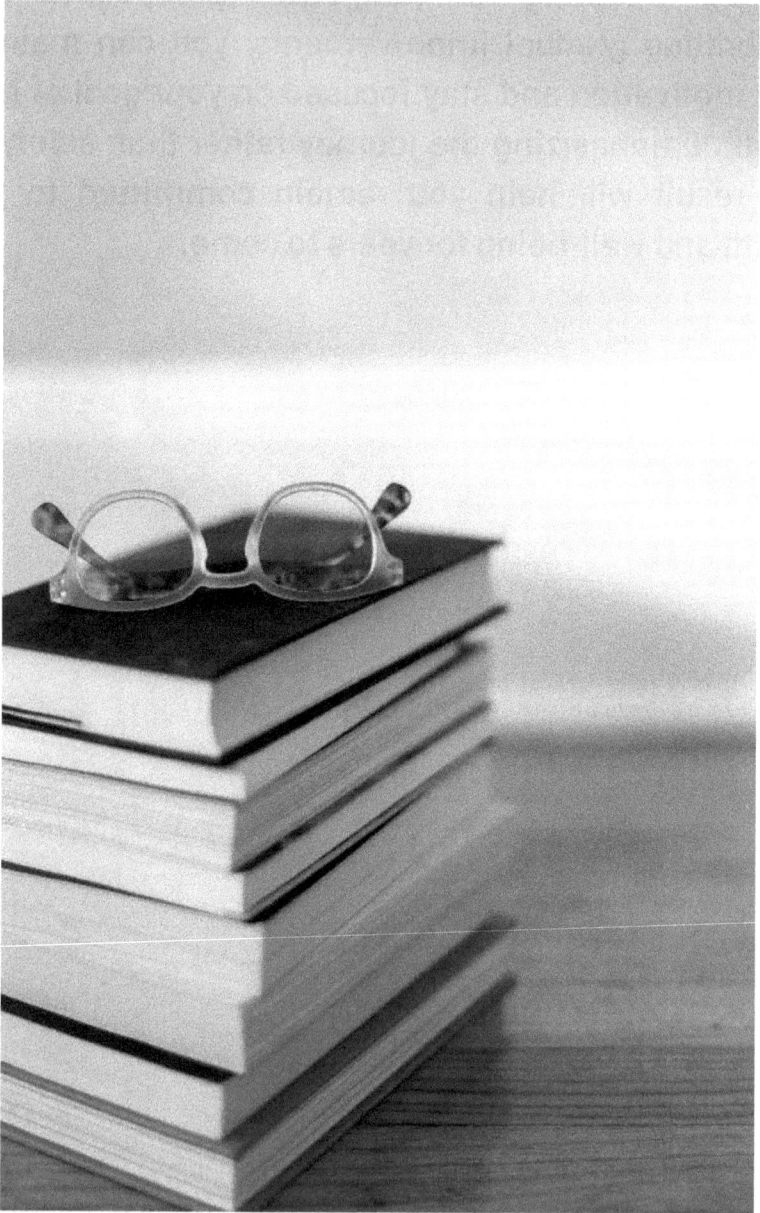

Chapter 13

Resources for Further Learning

Recommended Books and Articles

For individuals seeking to prevent coronary artery disease, a wealth of resources is available that can deepen understanding and provide practical strategies. One highly recommended book is "The Heart Health Bible" by Dr. Robert M. Ginsburg.

This comprehensive guide offers insight into heart health and emphasizes lifestyle changes that can significantly reduce the risk of coronary artery disease. Dr. Ginsburg's evidence-based approach, combined with easy-to-follow advice on diet, exercise, and stress management, makes it an essential read for anyone serious about heart health.

Another valuable resource is "Prevent and Reverse Heart Disease" by Dr. Caldwell B. Esselstyn Jr. This book presents compelling research on the impact of a plant-based diet in preventing and even reversing heart disease. Dr. Esselstyn shares personal accounts of patients who have successfully transformed their health through dietary changes, providing not only motivation but also practical meal plans and recipes. This resource is particularly useful for readers looking to make significant dietary changes that can lead to improved heart health.

In addition to books, various articles in reputable medical journals and health magazines can offer current insights and research findings related to coronary artery disease prevention. For instance, articles published in journals like the Journal of the American College of Cardiology and Circulation provide peer-reviewed studies that explore the latest advancements in heart disease research. These articles often focus on emerging risk factors, innovative treatment options, and the role of genetics in heart health, making them invaluable for those who wish to stay informed about the latest developments in the field.

Furthermore, lifestyle magazines such as "Prevention" and "Health" frequently feature articles specifically focused on heart health and disease prevention. These publications often include expert interviews, personal success stories, and practical tips that are easily applicable to daily life. Readers can find guidance on topics such as heart-healthy cooking, effective exercise routines, and stress reduction techniques, all of which are crucial for maintaining a healthy heart and preventing coronary artery disease.

For those who prefer digital resources, numerous websites and online platforms offer a wealth of information on coronary artery disease prevention. The American Heart Association and the National Heart, Lung, and Blood Institute provide access to articles, toolkits, and research summaries that can help individuals understand the importance of prevention strategies. Engaging with these resources can empower readers to take proactive steps towards a healthier lifestyle and ultimately reduce their risk of coronary artery disease.

Online Resources and Communities

Online resources and communities play a crucial role in the prevention of coronary artery disease (CAD) by providing education, support, and motivation to individuals seeking to improve their heart health. The internet offers a vast array of websites, forums, and social media platforms dedicated to heart health, where users can access up-to-date information on risk factors, lifestyle modifications, and the latest research findings.

Websites maintained by reputable health organizations, such as the American Heart Association and the Centers for Disease Control and Prevention, offer evidence based guidelines and recommendations that can empower individuals to make informed decisions about their health.

In addition to official health websites, online communities provide a platform for individuals to connect with others who share similar goals and challenges. These communities can be found on social media platforms, blogs, and dedicated health forums.

Engaging with others who are also interested in preventing CAD can foster a sense of belonging, encourage accountability, and provide emotional support. Sharing personal experiences, tips, and success stories can motivate individuals to stay committed to their goals and inspire them to adopt healthier lifestyles.

Webinars, online courses, and virtual workshops are also valuable resources for those looking to deepen their understanding of heart health. Many organizations offer free or low-cost educational programs that cover topics such as nutrition, exercise, stress management, and smoking cessation.

These resources often feature expert speakers, interactive discussions, and the opportunity to ask questions, making them an excellent way to gain knowledge and practical skills necessary for preventing CAD. Participating in these online events can enhance an individual's ability to implement lifestyle changes effectively.

Moreover, mobile applications focused on health and fitness have become increasingly popular tools for monitoring and improving heart health. These apps can help users track their physical activity, dietary habits, and vital health metrics like blood pressure and cholesterol levels. Some applications also offer personalized workout plans and meal suggestions tailored to individual health goals.

By utilizing technology, individuals can gain insights into their progress and receive reminders to stay on track, making it easier to maintain a heart-healthy lifestyle.

Finally, online resources can also aid in identifying local support groups or health programs that complement digital engagement. Many communities offer virtual meetings or hybrid options for those unable to attend in person. These groups often provide a structured environment for discussing challenges, sharing resources, and celebrating successes.

By combining online and local resources, individuals can create a comprehensive support system that reinforces their commitment to preventing coronary artery disease and achieving long-term heart health.

Professional Organizations and Support Groups

Professional organizations and support groups play a crucial role in the prevention and management of coronary artery disease (CAD). These entities provide valuable resources, education, and support for individuals seeking to reduce their risk of developing heart-related issues.

Many organizations are dedicated to heart health, offering a wealth of information on lifestyle changes, nutritional guidance, and exercise programs that can significantly impact cardiovascular well-being.

One of the most prominent organizations in this field is the American Heart Association (AHA). The AHA offers comprehensive resources, including research findings, guidelines for healthy living, and access to local community events focused on heart health. Their initiatives promote awareness of heart disease risk factors and emphasize the importance of regular check-ups and screenings.

By engaging with such organizations, individuals can stay informed about the latest advancements in CAD prevention and connect with professionals who can guide them through the process.

Support groups are another essential component of the CAD prevention landscape. These groups provide a platform for individuals to share their experiences, challenges, and successes in managing their heart health. Connecting with others facing similar struggles fosters a sense of community and accountability. Support groups often host meetings featuring guest speakers, health professionals, and nutritionists who can offer practical advice on lifestyle modifications.

Participants can learn from one another, gain motivation, and develop strategies to tackle the challenges of preventing coronary artery disease.

In addition to local support groups, online forums and virtual communities have gained popularity, especially in recent years. These platforms allow individuals to connect with peers from around the world, share resources, and access information at their convenience.

Online support groups often provide anonymity, making it easier for individuals to discuss sensitive topics related to heart health without fear of judgment. This accessibility ensures that a broader audience can benefit from the collective knowledge and experiences of others, regardless of their geographic location.

Finally, healthcare providers often collaborate with professional organizations and support groups to enhance patient care. By integrating the resources available through these entities into their practice, healthcare professionals can offer a more holistic approach to CAD prevention.

Patients are encouraged to take an active role in their health by leveraging these resources, which can lead to improved outcomes. Engaging with professional organizations and support groups is an effective way for individuals to empower themselves in the journey toward preventing coronary artery disease.

Author Notes & Acknowledgments

First and foremost, I would like to express my deepest gratitude to the people who inspired and supported me throughout the journey of writing this book. This project would not have been possible without their unwavering belief in me and their invaluable contributions.

To my wife, thank you for your constant encouragement and understanding. Your love and support have been my anchor during the challenging times of researching and writing this book. Your belief in my ability to make a difference in people's lives has been my driving force.

I would also like to disclose that this book contains some renewed artificial intelligence-generated content. I really appreciate very recent technological innovation by outstanding scientists and of course our reader's understanding.

Lastly, I want to express my deepest gratitude to the readers of this book. I sincerely hope the strategies and methods outlined within these pages will provide you with the knowledge and tools needed to truly make your life much better. Your commitment to seeking any good solutions and willingness to explore multiple methods is commendable.

Author Bio

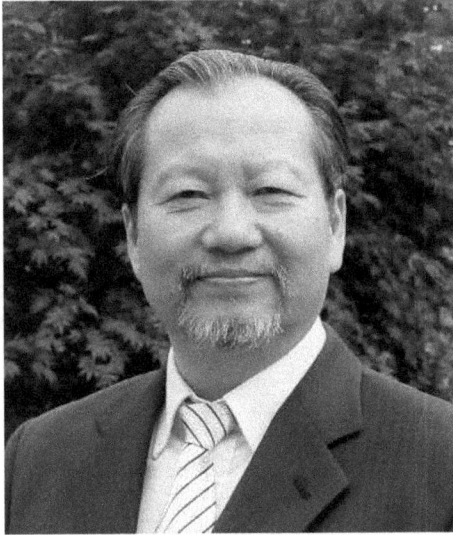

Johnson Wu earned his MD in 1982. With over 40 years of clinical experience, he has worked in hospitals in Zhejiang and Shanghai, China, as well as the Royal Marsden Hospital (part of Imperial College) in London, UK. Upon the recommendation of Sir Aaron Klug, the president of The Royal Society and a Nobel Prize winner in Chemistry, Dr. Wu was honorably awarded a British Royal Society Fellowship. He has published over 100 medical books in many countries and currently practices medicine in Canada.